What Your Vet
Never Told You

Secrets to Supporting Peak Health
for Your Animal

What Your Vet Never Told You

Secrets to Supporting Peak Health for Your Animal

Odette Suter, DVM

www.PeakAnimalHealthCenter.com
661-993-1979

Dedication

To all animals and people who enrich this beautiful planet with their hearts.

Acknowledgments

My entire life has been blessed with amazing people and animals—alive and in spirit form. They are my teachers and companions on this wild journey into the depth of healing. Without all of them my life would not be what it is now. They have made it possible for this book to be created. Each one has led me a step further into what I didn't know existed, but deeply desired.

My wonderful parents instilled curiosity and a deep respect for nature and our planet. They taught me to look beyond the apparent and supported me so generously to follow my soul's calling. Thank you for nurturing my soul and giving me the best start in life.

To my best friend and sister, Fabienne: I could not live this life without you!

A special thank you to my *adoptive parents* as I call them, Ann and Huug. They have shared my love for animals and have always picked me up when I needed it.

Along my journey I have met many teachers who have given of themselves so generously:

Jakob Oeler, my first riding instructor and someone I think of as my grandfather;

Dr. Hiltrud Strasser, who blew my mind wide open;

Penelope Smith, whose teaching unlocked the piece of my heart that yearned to be even closer to my animal friends;

Esther Ting, LAc, who taught me how to be more at peace with what is;

Dr. Kerry Ridgway, who took me under his wing;

Biochemist Linsey McLean, who shared her knowledge so generously;

and Dr. Carl DeStefano, who encouraged me to not give up, to keep going until I found an answer.

Thanks to Drs. Margo Roman, Pedro Rivera, W. Jean Dodds, Alan Schoen, and all fellow holistic veterinarians for the knowledge shared and contributed to our profession. Thanks to all my colleagues, who support me like a family.

In addition to many teachers who have provided bits and pieces of education, I would like to thank all the people and animals who have come to me for help. You have challenged me to go further than I thought possible.

To my family and friends, whose unconditional love and support over the years is gratefully received and returned a hundredfold.

To my book mentors, for giving me the tools and support to write this book and get it published. I would especially like to thank Maura, Keith, Amy, Heather, and everyone at YouSpeakIt Books Program who has helped bring this book to fruition. It is with their experience and expertise that I've been able to write this book and bring this information to animal lovers. Thank you for your contributions, hard work, and dedication.

To everyone reading this book and allowing me to share my knowledge with you, thank you for your help in sharing my mission to end suffering.

I have been truly blessed with a passion for healing and Oneness. Thank you Great Spirit for guiding my life so perfectly and for loving me.

Contents

Introduction

Why is your animal sick?

Why?

There is always a reason for your animal's state of health — It's up to you to find it.

Why is the most important question to ask.

Children ask this question all the time.

Why do we ask why when our car breaks down, but we don't ask why when our animals' bodies don't work as they should?

Why do our animals have so many illnesses?

- Obesity
- Allergies
- Cancer
- Anxiety
- Hormone imbalance
- Lethargy
- Recurrent infections

A lot of good information is available to us for keeping the animals in our lives in the best of well-being. However, it is hard to wade through it all and get a good overview of what it takes to keep an animal healthy or help it return to vibrant health.

This book has many purposes:

- To help you answer why
- To empower you to know more
- To help you take good care of your animals
- To provide animals with a healthy and happy life
- To show you how to prevent disease and suffering for your animals
- To teach you that improving your animal's health can improve your own health and life

I tried for years to improve my health, which was compromised by autoimmune challenges, such as chronic fatigue syndrome and all its unpleasantness. It's taken me years to get my health back and if I had known then what I know now, it would have been a much shorter journey. I want to share what I have learned along the path.

I want to make this journey shorter for everyone, especially for your animals because they don't live as long as we do; they don't have as much time. I want to provide you with as much information as possible in order to create a faster healing journey.

Many people turn to holistic medicine after having exhausted a traditional approach, but holistic medicine is unfortunately often used like traditional allopathic medicine. Instead of using drugs, it uses herbs and other natural treatments to chase after and treat isolated symptoms. Used this way, it is just as ineffectual as allopathic medicine, because it's not addressing the cause of the issue; it's just treating symptoms. A healthcare provider is practicing true holistic medicine only when they approach healing in consideration of the whole being.

Doing a little bit here and a little bit there won't get you the results that you're looking for. If a dog is aggressive, for example, relying on training alone to get the aggression under control may only work to a certain extent. It will not work to the degree that you would hope, because there's potentially another issue underneath—such as hypothyroidism—that needs to be addressed.

Health concerns are often much more complex than we think. Diseases typically are not just back pain, a little bit of limping somewhere, or an ear infection. Usually there are more factors involved. We need to look at the whole animal, not its symptoms alone. As a veterinarian, when I was addressing only the little bits and pieces rather than the whole animal, I felt like I was working with my hands tied behind my back.

Allow your veterinarian to take care of your animal's entire being, and you will see much greater changes.

Following that logic, I would encourage you to read this entire book in sequence for the best results. I advise against doing a little bit of detox here, a little bit of exercise there, or a little bit of hormone therapy standing alone. Read the book as a whole, and look at its suggestions as a whole. Address your animal's health using *all* of the information rather than just a part. You will get much faster and better results that way.

Finding a mentor is very much part of regaining good health. Don't try to do it all by yourself; find someone; work with someone. You may have to invest a little bit of money, but you will get better results with someone in your corner who is more experienced than you are than if you just fiddle around by yourself. You wouldn't learn to pilot a plane by yourself; you'd have to have a mentor. The same is true for your animal's health.

I also urge you to take action. Don't procrastinate. Once you have a sense of where you need to go, take one small step at a time, so it won't seem overwhelming. Develop a plan of manageable steps. Seek help to do this effectively. Please connect with me via email or phone.

I hope that reading this helps you to gain a different understanding of how animal (and human) bodies work, how our environment affects and supports us, and what we need to do to keep our animals healthy. I'm also hoping that you gain relief. Information is available for whatever issues you and your animals may be dealing with.

This book conveys the message that even though we live in a world with much pain and suffering, there is hope. If you know what is going on, then you can do something about it. This book empowers you. It's about changing our whole healthcare system and how that system is used. Help me spread the word about what's possible and how things are. Share what you're learning from this book with others whose animals are sick.

At the end of each section you'll find information on specific actions you can take to improve your animal's health.

Enjoy the book! Learn from it, and have an open mind as you're reading it.

CHAPTER ONE

The Value of Animals and the Cost of Disease

Until one has loved an animal,
a part of one's soul remains unawakened.

~ Anatole France

MY STORY: FINDING MY PATH

Animals have been a part of my life ever since my early childhood. Although I didn't have much of a connection to our guinea pig, Penelope (I always had to clean her cage), some others slowly infiltrated my heart and guided me on my journey to becoming a veterinarian.

One experience in particular was instrumental in the revelation that I would be a veterinarian; it wasn't even a choice. A thoroughbred horse named Conifer had fallen and injured both *carpi*, or what we think of as the knees on a horse. He needed stitches to close the wounds on his knees.

When the vet came, I remember him kneeling beside the horse. I watched as he sutured the skin back together. I was on the other side of the horse and I couldn't take my eyes off the procedure. I was really surprised that I didn't want to turn away. Somehow it didn't faze me much.

The whole experience felt a bit surreal to me. It was like when something happens and you are removed from it. My wiser soul pushed my conscious, logical, thinking brain out of the way so I could take in what was happening without getting confused by emotions or mental chatter.

It's difficult to put into words, but it felt like an intervention of sorts, like when you wake up from a dream and think: *was that really real?*

In that moment, Destiny took me by the hand and gave me a really strong message from my soul to pursue a path of veterinary medicine.

Now when I work as a vet, I still feel that force. It's as if the healing comes from some other place. To this day, every time an animal gets better through my assistance, I'm still in awe of the body's ability to heal and by the miracle of healing.

It's funny how my life unfolded. I dreamed I would have a big farm in France with lots of animals, but Spirit had other plans. Today it is not at all what I thought it would be. Everything turned out very differently, and much better, than I imagined.

My first teachers were my mother and father. They raised me in a very natural, holistic sort of way. They encouraged me to learn about herbs, organic gardening, and leading a healthy lifestyle. Their guidance shaped my path.

I learned from my parents to have an open mind, and I find that is one of the most important qualities of being a veterinarian. While I was a student I worked as a hoof-care practitioner, trimming horses' hooves. One of the ponies I was taking care of at the time suffered from a sinus infection that just wouldn't heal despite the most up-to-date treatments at the equine hospital. Since nothing seemed to be working, the pony's guardian contacted a psychic.

I remember exactly the thoughts that were running through my head; just like everyone else, I thought: *this is crazy and it won't work.*

But a little voice in my head instructed me: *Be open, because who knows? Maybe this psychic really is onto something.*

She was.

What she found ended up being quite true, and her recommendation helped heal that pony. My whole mind changed again. I was more open to new ideas and new things.

Every time since then when something different has presented itself, it has turned into a good thing. New ideas and experiences have led me in a direction that was meant to be and has trained me to be the veterinarian that I am today.

Another big part of my education has been through my own healing journey. Even though I grew up living in a very healthy way, my physical constitution wasn't as strong as I would have liked.

My body took on a lot of stress caused by several life events:

- My mother's passing
- Veterinary school and exams
- Stepping into the world as a veterinarian

Those stressors caused me to become quite sick. I ended up with chronic fatigue syndrome. For a long time I could barely move. I didn't have any energy; I was just lying on my sofa all day doing nothing.

I tried many different modalities to heal myself and take my energy back:

- Acupuncture
- Herbs
- Chiropractic care
- Detox
- Hormones
- Massage
- Reiki
- Cranio-sacral therapy
- Meditation
- Homeopathy
- Bio-resonance
- Nutraceuticals
- Neurotransmitter therapy

I didn't leave any stone unturned, and with each stone I did overturn, I learned a lot more. Sometimes I was exposed to a whole different philosophy of healing. Every step took me deeper into what healing is and what disease is.

I've had many mentors on the way that have contributed. Each one has taught me something different, and shown me how to look at life in a different way and open my heart to more than what I knew. They taught me to be courageous and brave and leap into the unknown.

My healing story didn't really end with that. Later on, I ended up with an autoimmune disease. It really taught me that if I wanted to heal my body even more,

I needed to address all the parts together, and that is what this book is about.

On my healing journey, I have learned that trying to heal one aspect of my body at a time does not work. I had to look at the health of my body as a whole system. As a result of this deep learning, I apply this to my healing work with animals.

Animals have been some of my greatest teachers, especially when I learned to listen to them more consciously. It confirmed what I already knew in my heart: that they are really our equals.

They have souls.

They talk to hearts.

They have feelings.

If we listen to them, we can hear their wisdom.

Animals are just as important as any human or any other living being. They have the same physical, emotional, and spiritual needs that we do. Animals can touch our hearts much more deeply than most humans can because animals don't judge us.

Their health also affects us very deeply. If they're not healthy or not enjoying life as much as we think they should, we suffer with them. Sometimes we end up suffering even more than they do, because in a way, they *are* our hearts.

ANIMALS ARE JUST LIKE US

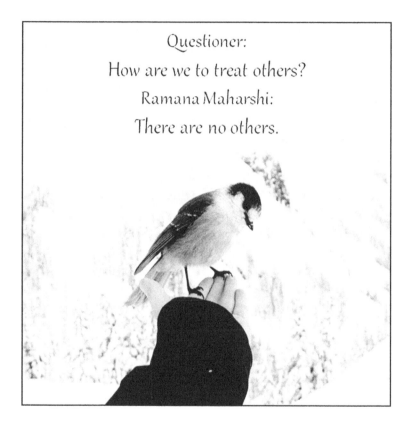

Questioner:
How are we to treat others?
Ramana Maharshi:
There are no others.

Bigger-Brained Humans: Are We Really Superior?

Many humans think that animals are less important than we are. Many cultures still believe that. Obviously, if you're reading this book, you probably are not among them.

Nevertheless, sometimes when I work with clients, I hear them say, "Well, I can't spend more money on my animal than myself."

Sometimes people tell me, "It is just an animal, after all."

Beliefs like these are still ingrained in our society, even if we love our animals very deeply.

We look at animals as pets. But still, many people act and behave as though they believe animals are inferior and deserve less than humans do. It's true that animals don't talk like we do. They don't express themselves like we do, so we assume their intelligence is less than ours.

They just have a different kind of intelligence. One that surpasses ours in some ways. Animals don't get distracted by everything in life as we do. They live in the moment and in their hearts, and that makes them indispensable to us. They remind us of who we are and what life is about.

A dog comes running at you wagging her tail, a big smile on her face. Your heart lights up; your life lights up. These are the reminders that they give us. They are with us every step of the way, supporting us. We can't be without them. As humans, we cannot be without animals, period. We would not be able to survive.

Animal Intelligence

When I first moved to the United States, I lived in a household with many animals. One of them was an orange tabby cat named Sherman, and he was certainly very smart. He was the guardian of emotions, I could say. If I was having a hard time, he would show up, and if I was having a hard time and he didn't show up, I knew whatever was troubling me wasn't really that bad. I was younger at the time, and I went through emotional difficulties more often. I could always count on Sherman to be a barometer of how much help I really needed in the moment.

One night, I was by myself. I heard this constant chirping that was very loud and piercing. I didn't know what it was, but I knew the house I was living in had some pipes going from a flat roof down through the house and probably draining water into something, somewhere. I thought there was a frog stuck in the pipe, so the next day, I went up there and looked at it. I couldn't hear or find anything, and tried to flush the pipe with water.

The next night, as I was trying to sleep, I was rather stressed out and not in the best of moods. The chirping continued as I was trying to sleep. Sherman didn't leave my side for a second. Every time that I moved, he would move too, so that he could be touching me again. That noise was very piercing, so obviously, for a cat a noise like that is even worse.

To make a long story short, the sound was coming from a smoke detector with a low battery. I didn't know about smoke detectors; I had just moved to the United States and we didn't have them in Switzerland.

So I changed the battery and everything was fine again. But it just shows that Sherman the Cat knew that I needed him because that noise was driving me crazy.

Animals Share Valuable Wisdom and Intuition

When I lived with Sherman, I was training in acupuncture. He was definitely a great teacher for me, because he was holding the space while I was practicing. A couple of times, he actually jumped on the table and pulled out one of the needles I had put into a patient. He knew that it had been in long enough to do its work and was no longer needed.

Of course, it about gave me a heart attack because I didn't want him to swallow the needle. He definitely trained me to be a little more attentive and feeling the energies a little bit more, so that I could do what *felt* right, rather than thinking with my head only. He trained me to be more sensitive and more in tune with what I was doing with the animal I was treating.

Every animal leads a life that we humans don't really know a whole lot about.

We only see:

- They're furry creatures.
- They're happy when they see us.
- They demand we fulfill their basic needs.

Animals are very important in many ways. Our pets support us on an emotional level, they're our friends, and they love us. At the same time, they love us while our wild counterparts fulfill different but equally important roles in our interconnected lives.

A great documentary was made about the wolves returning to Yellowstone Park. These wolves restored the entire ecosystem there to be much healthier. Their presence had a big impact on the environment. It rebuilt the natural environment, rebalanced it, and eventually changed the flow of the rivers.

Even a slug, tick, or mosquito has a role in our ecosystem, and it would be wise for us to respect and love all of them for what they are and what they bring. If there were no bees, for example, we would be missing some vital pollinators. Our food, flowers, and any products related to fruiting plants would suffer.

We are not in any way, shape, or form more important than any animal, be it a big or a small animal. Humanity with all its so-called intelligence has created so much damage that we are a much bigger threat to this planet than any other animal ever could be. Animals deserve just as much, or more, respect as we do.

COST VERSUS INVESTMENT

This book is not only about our animals. It's also about us, because we are connected. Humans and animals live together. We share life together. Any time one of your animals isn't doing as well as it should, it affects your life on many levels. We don't like to see our animals suffer; we suffer almost more than they do when they're sick.

But there's much more to a cat, dog, or horse than meets the eye. Many people have learned that, especially when they needed a good friend or when they needed love. Horses were like friends to me when I was growing up. They were my confidants. I could talk to them about anything. I didn't actually say anything to them; they just knew what was going on, and they would hold the space and love me. Animals have done that for me my entire life, more than any human could have done.

Animal Wellness Affects Our Emotions and Relationships

I know that many of you experience this too. Animals enrich your life so much. The bond goes both ways: When your animal feels good, you feel good. When they are hurt or unwell, you also feel unwell. When your animal is sick, you probably feel stressed yourself.

You may find that helping your injured or ill animal also affects your relationships, because the stress you experience is transmitted into the relationships closest to you; in particular, into those at work, with friends, and so on.

Many people who come to me say, "I cannot leave my animal alone! I can't go on vacation. I cannot go out because of my animal needs my help."

That creates a lot of stress, unhappiness, and sickness for ourselves, too. It's a bit like compassion fatigue in people who take care of a loved one with Alzheimer's, for example.

And what if your partner or other family members aren't on the same page as you?

They want to travel and all you want to do is stay home with your beloved furry friend. When your animal is not healthy, it can affect you greatly in that respect. It could limit how you experience life and the joy that you could have.

As a veterinarian, I see the pain my clients carry. It breaks my heart. When animals are not healthy it affects pretty much everybody who is in their lives.

The Financial Effects

The financial burden of having a sick animal is considerable. Sadly, disease can end in premature euthanasia, because the cost of treatment is beyond financial means.

Added to the pain of losing an animal can be heavy feelings of guilt and what we call "should haves":

I should have noticed something sooner.

I should have acted sooner.

When you're faced with a life-and-death decision, choosing life can take a big chunk of money out of your bank account. Medical cost is the number one cause of bankruptcy.

Prevention is a lot less costly on all levels. If you don't take care of your animals preventatively, you may end up paying a very high price. Procrastinating preventive care is not a good idea. You may pay a little more up front, but the cost of an animal being sick is much higher. Not to mention that once the emergency has passed, the animal is usually not healthier than before; it is often worse off. Thus, using money for prevention is an investment in their health that will pay back in dividends for years to come.

Nico, a cat, is a perfect example of how illness can become costly if we don't fix the underlying cause. Nico was suffering from recurrent pancreatic inflammation, which required frequent hospitalization. He was reacting to most kinds of protein except duck and lamb. Food sensitivity was causing constant inflammation in his gut including an imbalance of his gastro-intestinal microbes.

Due to the proximity to the pancreas and liver, both these organs can be affected. Pancreatitis and chronic liver problems often go hand in hand with small intestinal issues. As a result, these animals can have significant discomfort, pain, and often end up in the hospital because they stop eating. Not only was Nico suffering from this kind of painful, internal inflammation, but the food sensitivities also manifested as skin problems.

His guardian writes:

> *You saved him – he almost died a couple of times! He was not having a very good quality of life. He had sores all over his body, he had inflamed ears, he was in pain and we tried everything that we could through conventional medicine . . . and if what you were offering wasn't going to fix him, I didn't think anything would.*
>
> *He has responded so well. He has no sores on his body. His ears are so much better. He's playing. He's normal. He's doing really, really well! The whole program was really helpful for everybody. Thank you!*
>
> — Mary D.

Questions and Action Steps

Many people tell me that their animals are their life.

What does your animal bring to your life?

How is it special?

CHAPTER TWO

What Does It Take to Be Healthy?

There's nothing more important than our good health –
that's our principal capital asset.

~ Arlen Specter

WHAT ARE HEALTH AND DISEASE?

When I was in veterinary school, the definition of *disease* was never really discussed. We learned about different diseases, but nobody ever really defined disease. I think it's important to look at what disease means and establish some good definitions. Developing this clarity will help pave the way to knowing what you need to do.

In our society, we're very quick to see symptoms, and we want to label these symptoms right away, because uncertainty is difficult to deal with. It's much harder to take a step back for a broader view of what is really going on. If you are like most of the population, you want a quick fix. You want to know what the disease is, and then you want to have the solution right away to end your animal's suffering.

There Is Only One Disease

There are a seemingly infinite number of diseases, and it is possible for your animal to have multiple diseases at the same time. While this is true, it is also possible to view all disease through a much simpler lens.

A broader definition of disease is *a malfunctioning of cells.*

Our bodies and our animals' bodies are made up of specialized cells that have different functions:

- Pancreas cells help regulate blood sugar levels.

- Cells in the gut govern how much nutrition is gained from food and liquid (among many other functions).

- Thyroid cells produce hormones that control all metabolic functions and the speed at which all biochemical reactions in the body occur.

If your animal has diabetes, for instance, you know that the cells of the pancreas are malfunctioning. If your animal has hypothyroidism, you know thyroid cells are having trouble. Understanding which cells are challenged gives you a lot of information about how to proceed.

However, no matter what kind of cell you're working with, the underlying principle of how to address the malfunction is the same.

The next question then becomes clear: "Why are these cells malfunctioning?"

This *why* is really the most important question. It is one that children ask all the time.

"Why is the sky blue?"

You give them an answer and they still ask why. Like most adults, you may have lost the childlike drive to relentlessly question why. You may want to get things over with as quickly as possible.

Take some time to engage in the process of asking these fundamental questions:

- Why do the cells malfunction?
- Why is disease present?
- Why do your animals not appear to feel well?
- What are their symptoms showing you?

These are the questions you need to ask, not, "What shampoo should I use for my dog's allergies?"

In this instance, the better questions to ask would be larger questions about the origin of allergy symptoms: "Why is my dog having an allergic reaction?"

The answer to the question of why cells malfunction is very simple. There can be two main causes: *deficiency* and *toxicity*.

Deficiency: the body is not getting the nutrients that it needs in order to be functioning properly.

Toxicity: something is interfering with the cells' ability to do their job.

For example, if you look at a wilted plant, what is your first thought?

It is missing something.

It needs some water, right?

Then, it might also need sunshine and nutrients.

What could be interfering with a plant's health to make it wilt?

Maybe it has a bug infestation, or somebody poured gasoline on it—something toxic—and so it gets sick from that.

This is really logical thinking, isn't it?

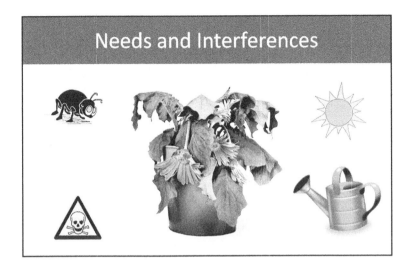

Needs and Interferences

Signs of Health, Signs of Disease

You probably think that you know what disease looks like.

Am I right?

I emphasize what health is—something that seems so logical—based on many experiences, such as the following:

A dog was brought to me for fly-biting behavior. The condition had been well controlled with seizure medication until it resurfaced with a vengeance after the dog was given a cocktail of drugs (heartworm preventative and tick/flea medicine) and vaccines (rabies and lepto). All of these preventative treatments can have a significant effect on the nervous system and body overall. They should not be given to a sick animal, especially not one with neurological issues. Because this dog hadn't shown any obvious symptoms at that time, he had been considered healthy. But any animal who is receiving treatment for any condition is still considered sick. This goes for animals with allergies, GI upset, or low thyroid, and so on.

You may be someone who knows what disease looks like, but many people—sadly, including some of my colleagues—will give preventative treatments to sick animals.

Behavioral issues can also result from a physical issue and should be considered as one until proven otherwise.

Signs of health include:

- Bright eyes
- Appropriate and balanced behavior
- Healthy skin and normal shedding of coat
- Optimal digestion
- Sound movement
- Well-developed muscles
- Strong tendons and ligaments
- Size-appropriate weight

These may be very logical to you, but often I hear:

"My dog is aggressive."

"My horse is lazy."

"It must be his or her personality."

"She's depressed."

"He's grumpy."

To me, those are actually signs of disease, because a healthy animal is a happy animal. Any time there is disease or feeling unwell, usually that manifests on an emotional level. Of course, there are some times where animals will behave inappropriately because of their life experiences, but if an animal isn't behaving normally, you need to look at what's going on physically.

The horse, Quito, is a perfect example. When I first met him he was always grumpy, hated to be groomed, and didn't have much energy. He was labeled as being lazy and cranky and in need of correction. But this poor horse was just not feeling well. He had stomach and intestinal ulcers that created pain and discomfort. Once his body healed, he was a completely different horse.

Signs of disease include:

- Dull eyes
- Inappropriate and imbalanced behavior ("lazy")

- Skin issues: slow shedding of coat, excessive coat growth
- GI problems: vomiting, abnormal feces
- Lameness
- Sore and poorly developed muscles
- Weak tendons and ligaments
- Obesity or low weight
- Respiratory issues

Here are a few examples of symptoms that are commonly ignored or misinterpreted:

- Hormonal imbalances can show up with shedding or excessive coat growth.

- Abnormal stool consistency — such as fecal water, diarrhea, or constipation — are signs that should not be ignored. Even if, for example, a horse defecates and there's just a little bit of water coming out, that is a sign that there may be something wrong in their GI tract.

- If your animal is limping, stiff, or has a hard time getting up (or getting up on the couch), or performing the way you would expect it to perform, that is a sign of an issue as well.

- Sore and poorly developed muscles can go hand in hand with GI issues. Sore backs due to GI issues are the norm.

- Although overfeeding leads to weight gain, I have found that weight issues are more related to other physical issues, such as a hormonal imbalance or inflammation in the GI tract.

- A dog who is eating socks and other inedible objects might have an underlying issue such as *rabies vaccinosis*, which is an adverse reaction to rabies vaccination.

We Have Everything We Need to Heal

When your animal is ill, think of its body as having some kind of impairment to healthy function, or lacking something. It could be both. Once you arrive at that conclusion, you will find that there is a lot you can do to help.

The fear-based system we live in tells us there is no solution or that we don't have enough knowledge. But we do know enough; the principle is simple: you need to provide the body what it requires and remove what it does not. There is enough information already available about what it takes to achieve this. If we were to actually apply the information available to us, we could end the epidemic of chronic disease!

You and your veterinarian don't really need to throw a lot of drugs or intensive research at a given issue to try to resolve it. Of course more research will always bring more insight into what's going on and how you can help. But you don't have to wait for billion-dollar research. You just have to change the way you think. To see the solution, you have to think outside of the box of the traditional medical system.

THE STRAW THAT BROKE THE CAMEL'S BACK

You may think: *Oh, my animal just came down with something. The symptom just showed up. He was healthy yesterday, now he is sick.*

Disease doesn't usually work that way.

Let me ask you this very important question: what are symptoms really?

Let's consider this analogy: what does it mean when the "check engine" light of your car is lit?

There is something wrong with the engine, right?

What does it mean if your animal has a symptom?

Something is wrong with the body.

Going back to the "check engine" light, does it light up because there is something wrong with the light itself?

No — it's not the light causing a problem; it's the engine.

The same is true for the body. Symptoms are simply a sign that there is an underlying problem. The symptom itself is just pointing to that problem and isn't usually the problem itself.

That's crucial to understand! Because if you do, you'll understand that a new shampoo or Benadryl will not stop your dog's skin allergies. If you stop treatment, the symptoms will be right back. It would be like covering the check engine light with a piece of tape. The problem is still there.

The Body Can Compensate for Only So Long

The body has an ability to compensate. As long as there are enough cells functioning properly, you won't see problems. But once the scale tips or the last straw has broken the camel's back, so to speak, you instantly see signs. Usually by this time, it's been developing for a very long while underneath the surface, a bit like a volcano that hasn't erupted yet. That's really how symptoms appear. When you see symptoms in an animal, they show you only the tip of the iceberg. They're simply signs that the animal has already been losing its health for some time.

Listen to the Symptoms; Don't Wait

If you see the tip of the iceberg, you had better respond to the symptoms. You need to take care of what you can't see under the surface.

As an example, let's look at what's going on when an animal has allergies. You have to find out what the cause is. When an animal is showing symptoms, usually there's inflammation present. If inflammation persists, it will slowly destroy other organs — it will not just stay with the allergies.

My childhood dog, Windy, is a perfect example. She started having allergies when she was about six years old. Every year the period of allergy grew longer until they were causing her discomfort year-round. During that time, she also had to have her spleen removed. It had grown so big that it was pushing on the liver. The liver couldn't function any more. The spleen was removed and she did okay after that, but a few years later she started to develop mammary cancer. Then a few years later, she developed dementia.

All of these things may seem like they're totally unrelated: the allergies were affecting the skin, which has nothing to do with the spleen, mammary glands, and brain.

These are totally unrelated areas, right?

Whenever there is chronic inflammation, other organ systems will be affected. You really need to listen to these early symptoms—or even better: prevent them all together. Please take action right away. Don't wait, because if you do, you may end up with much bigger problems for your animal down the road that are much more difficult and costly to heal.

Your Actions Determine Your Animal's Health

Whatever you have done for your animal until now has determined their health up to this point. What you decide to do from now on really determines their health and their ability to enjoy life for months and years to come. A huge problem in our society–and I think you would probably agree with me—is that we tend to be procrastinators. We tend to put our animal's health (and our own) on the back burner, especially if it's not something we deem serious, and we wait until it hits us big-time to take action.

The fact that you're reading this book means that you're setting your animal's health as somewhat of a priority. But whether you're going to take action from this point on is really going to determine its health. If you want to make changes in your animal's health, you have to do something different. You have to make changes. You have to take action. It's much easier to take care of little symptoms as they show up, even taking care of preventing these little symptoms from showing up, than trying to fix something when the animal is close to being on its deathbed.

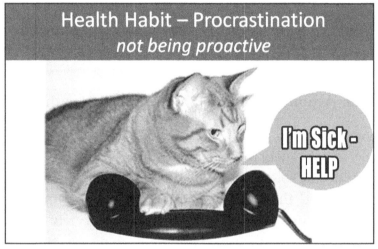

Symptoms are the body's call for help.

TIMES HAVE CHANGED

"But we've fed this for forty years and none of our previous animals had a problem."

Unfortunately our world has changed and not for the better. As a result things that once worked don't anymore. The reality is that our environment has changed and with every generation, health issues show up sooner and more frequently.

We need to be aware that our environment has changed tremendously in the past hundred years or so. Since World War II, 1.5 million new chemicals have been put on the market. Most of them are carcinogenic, and most of them have not been tested for safety.

Eighty thousand of these new chemicals, called *xenoestrogens*, interfere with hormones. They cause imbalance in the hormonal system, which leads to a lot of health issues. In addition, in the 1920s there were fewer than one million pounds of synthetic chemicals produced in the United States. In the year 2000, production exceeded 400 *billion* pounds. These chemicals aren't just sitting somewhere in a factory. They are being distributed in air, soil, and water all over the world. With this onslaught of chemicals, there's no way that the body can respond and cope the same way it had for centuries. It needs much more help to stay somewhat healthy.

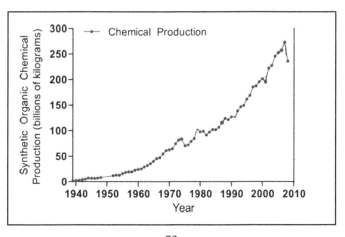

We're exposed to toxins everywhere, as are our animals:

- In the air from industrial exhaust (cars, planes, factories)
- In the water
- In the food
- In the drugs
- In the environment of our individual animals (such as fire retardants in the furniture)
- In the body products we use

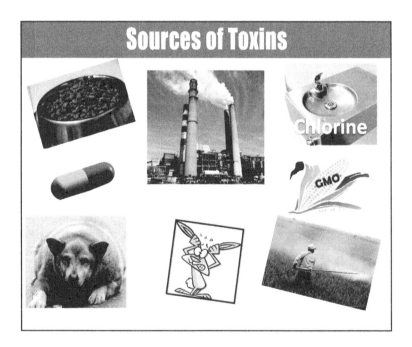

Bodies Cannot Detox Fast Enough

The body's detoxification system was made to deal with the waste that's being produced in the body from normal metabolism, and whatever might have come in food that was still relatively toxin-free. With the 140-billion-plus pounds of chemicals in our environment, the body becomes overloaded with toxins. Not only are there too many toxins for the detox pathways to be able to eliminate, but these toxins will also impair these detoxification pathways. The damage is twofold.

What about evolution?

Often I hear, "Well, our dogs have had kibble since the late 1800s; they should have adapted to that."

The truth is that the physiology of an animal, or a human, does not adapt to change that quickly. It took billions of years for the body to develop the way it is, and it's not going to change in one hundred years. All of our bodies are exposed to things they just can't handle.

Be Proactive

Based on what I just shared, doesn't it make sense that you need to be proactive, even if your animal is not showing any symptoms yet?

It's not a question of *if* your animal is going to get sick, it is probably more of a question of *when* your animal will be sick. Depending on its constitution and how healthy its ancestors were, your animal may not get sick until it's older. But we don't know. So I highly recommended taking action now, because procrastinating will most likely lead to disease.

We need to change our view and start to practice *health*-care, rather than *disease*-care. By healthcare I mean:

- Preventing issues
- Being proactive
- Helping the body to stay healthy

You've heard the adage: *An ounce of prevention is worth a pound of cure.*

If you prevent illness, you're investing money into your animals to keep them healthy. If they end up sick, it becomes a cost, be it financial or emotional. Find yourself a veterinarian who thinks proactively and who's interested in helping you do true prevention.

Questions and Action Steps

To get a better sense of your animal's health please check your animal's symptoms using the list that follows. You may be surprised about how many symptoms they actually had or currently have.

What drugs has your animal been on?

What toxins do you expose your animal to on a regular basis?

For instance, if you bathe them with a shampoo, look at the label. Choose a shampoo made of ingredients that you can pronounce and are nontoxic. Super hygiene is as prevalent for animals as it is for humans. Dirt is good. Dirt supplies the body with life-enhancing microbes. Every time we wash an animal with shampoo, we disturb the beneficial organisms and remove the protective layers.

The following is a list of symptoms and drugs adapted from *The Canine Thyroid Epidemic* by W. Jean Dodds and Diana R. Laverdure (Direct Book Service, 2011).

Reproductive disorders:

- ☐ Infertility
- ☐ Prolonged interestrus interval
- ☐ Lack of libido
- ☐ Absence of heat cycles
- ☐ Testicular atrophy
- ☐ Silent heats
- ☐ Hypospermia/aspermia
- ☐ Pseudopregnancy
- ☐ Weak, dying, or stillborn pups
- ☐ Poor growth

Behavioral issues:

- ☐ Depression
- ☐ Anxiety, irritability, aggression
- ☐ Lack of concentration
- ☐ Decreased ability to handle stress
- ☐ Whining
- ☐ Separation anxiety
- ☐ Fearfulness/nervousness
- ☐ Schizoid behavior
- ☐ Fear around strangers
- ☐ Hyperventilating
- ☐ Disorientation
- ☐ Moodiness
- ☐ Erratic temperament
- ☐ Hyperactivity

- □ Submissiveness
- □ Passivity
- □ Compulsiveness

Dermatologic diseases:

- □ Dry and thin skin
- □ Chronic offensive odor
- □ Coarse, dull coat
- □ Hair loss or excess hair growth
- □ Rat tail
- □ Puppy coat
- □ Seborrhea with greasy or dry skin
- □ Hyperpigmentation
- □ Pyoderma or skin infections

Immunologic disorders:

- □ Increased time to recover from illness or injury
- □ Immune deficiencies
- □ IgA deficiency
- □ Chronic infections
- □ Yeast overgrowth
- □ Allergies
- □ Hives
- □ Autoimmune diseases
- □ Cancer
- □ Sarcoids

Cardiovascular disorders:

- ☐ Slow heart rate
- ☐ Arrhythmias
- ☐ Cardiomyopathy

Hematologic (blood) disorders:

- ☐ Bleeding
- ☐ Bone marrow failure
- ☐ Low red blood cells, white blood cells, platelets

Occular diseases:

- ☐ Corneal lipid deposits
- ☐ Corneal ulceration
- ☐ Uveitis
- ☐ Dry eye
- ☐ Infections of eyelid glands

Other disorders:

- ☐ Loss of smell
- ☐ Loss of taste
- ☐ Glycosuria
- ☐ Chronic active hepatitis
- ☐ Diabetes
- ☐ Insulin resistance
- ☐ Vaccine reaction
- ☐ Infections

Gastrointestinal disorders:

- ☐ Constipation
- ☐ Diarrhea
- ☐ Vomiting
- ☐ Irritable bowel disease
- ☐ Ulcers

Alterations in cellular metabolism:

- ☐ Lethargy
- ☐ Weight gain/loss
- ☐ Mental dullness
- ☐ Cold intolerance
- ☐ Exercise intolerance
- ☐ Mood swings
- ☐ Seizures
- ☐ Polyneuropathy
- ☐ Hyperexcitability
- ☐ Chronic infections
- ☐ High cholesterol
- ☐ Liver disorders
- ☐ Low body temperature
- ☐ Slow metabolism

Neuromuscular and Skeletal problems:

- ☐ Weakness
- ☐ Knuckling or dragging feet

- Stiffness
- Muscle wasting
- Laryngeal paralysis
- Megoesophagus
- Facial paralysis
- Head tilt
- Tragic expression
- Drooping eyelids
- Incontinence
- Ruptured cruciate ligaments
- Other soft tissue damage
- Poor topline
- OCD lesion
- Laminitis/Founder
- Arthritis

Drugs Used:

- Antibiotics
- Non-steroidal anti-inflammatory drugs
- Antifungals
- Steroids
- Antihistamines
- Thyroid medication
- Chemotherapy agents
- Anti-parasitic drugs

CHAPTER THREE

The Limits of Our Healthcare System

America's healthcare system is neither healthy, caring, nor a system.
~ Walter Cronkite

You can't afford to get sick, and you can't depend on the present healthcare system to keep you well. It's up to you to protect and maintain your body's innate capacity for health and healing by making the right choices in how you live.
~ Andrew Weil

THE TRUTH ABOUT OUR HEALTHCARE SYSTEM

It's important to look closely at our healthcare system and know how it works in order to be able to figure out the best treatment for our animals. There are limitations in every healthcare system and every approach, and we need to know those in order to be able to make better choices.

Facts About Our Healthcare System

- **Noncommunicable diseases (e.g., chronic diseases) are the leading global causes of death, causing more deaths than all other causes combined . . . These diseases have reached epidemic proportions.** (www.who.int/nmh/publications/ncd_report_full_en.pdf)

- **Eighty-five percent of all medical procedures and surgeries are scientifically unproven.** (*British Medical Journal* 303:5 Oct., 1991)

- **In 2014, U.S. healthcare spending reached $3 trillion, or $9,523.00 per person.** (Centers for Medicare and Medicaid Services, www.cms.gov/Research-Statistics-Data-and-Systems/Statistics-Trends-and-Reports/NationalHealthExpendData/downloads/highlights.pdf).

- **Pharmaceutical companies spent more than $27 billion in advertising in 2012.** (www.skainfo.com/health_care_market_reports/2012_promotional_spending.pdf)

- **The U.S. medical system is the leading cause of death and injury in the United States.** (*Death by Medicine*, Gary Null, MD, Axios Press, 2011)

- **The U.S. healthcare system ranks thirty-seventh in the world, behind countries such as Saudi Arabia and Singapore.** (thepatientfactor. com/canadian-health-care-information/ world-health-organizations-ranking-of-the-worlds-health-systems/)

Today, more than 95 percent of all chronic disease is caused by food choice, toxic food ingredients, nutritional deficiencies, and lack of physical exercise.

~ Mike Adams

Similar tendencies are going on for animals. When I was in vet school we didn't see as many animals with cancer, autoimmune diseases, and other chronic diseases.

The occurrence of chronic diseases in pets has increased:

- Cancer
- Allergies
- Diabetes
- Arthritis
- Dental disease

Chronic diseases are the currently most prevalent.

In fact, Banfield Pet Hospital has pooled all of their data from 2006 to 2011 and they found increases in the following diseases:

Diabetes mellitus:

- Dogs 32 percent
- Cats 16 percent

Dental disease:

- Dog 12 percent
- Cats 10 percent

Otitis externa:

- Dogs 9 percent
- Cats 34 percent

Arthritis:

- Dogs 38 percent
- Cats 67 percent

Obesity:

- Dogs: 37 percent
- Cats: 90 percent

Kidney failure, allergies, hypothyroidism, and other illnesses are on the rise as well. Sadly, traditional medicine has very little to offer to treat these kinds of diseases. Most treatments cause significant side effects and certainly not a resolution of the issue.

A study by RT Branson regarding cancer revealed:

- Forty-five percent of dogs older than ten years die of cancer.

- One in four dogs develops a tumor during its lifetime.

- Cancer accounts for nearly 50 percent of all disease-related pet deaths each year.

First, we have to question what our healthcare system is really doing if it's not able to control these diseases.

Second, we have to figure out why there is such an increase. It's very unlikely for instance, that within five years people suddenly fed their cats so differently that double the number of cats suffers from obesity. That doesn't explain it; something must have happened on a larger scale.

Knowledge, Information, and Marketing

A foolish faith in authority is the worst enemy of truth.
                                    ~ Albert Einstein

Is there enough information available to you?

Is it clear information?

Is it information that's useful?

Can you trust that information?

I hear from animal owners that they are often confused by all the information that is available on the Internet. The truth is that it is confusing and it is difficult to know what to believe and what not to believe. In recent years, it has become clear that a lot of the scientific studies that are being done are fraudulent. Some are created out of the blue by the pharmaceutical industry or other entities that have a vested interest. That makes it difficult to know what is true and what isn't.

A lot of the information is also based on marketing.

What is in TV commercials?

It's quite crazy that drug ads list a whole slew of side effects, including *sudden death.* But their ads work! A lot of popular knowledge comes from their marketing.

If I start the sentence, you'll probably be able to finish it: "Milk, it _____." (does a body good)

Where does that information come from?

Who came up with it?

Was it the healthcare industry, or was it the milk industry?

Obviously, it was the milk industry because they want to sell their milk. Much of the information put into people's brains is pure marketing. We have to be aware of that, and be a little bit more discerning about what might be true and what might not be true. But it's not always easy. What we think is true today may turn out to be wrong tomorrow.

Cost Versus Investment

In my practice, I often see animals brought to me when their disease process is already far advanced. It breaks my heart. For that reason, I encourage people to be proactive and practice preventative care.

But often they tell me it's too expensive and they "can't feed that sort of food. Fifty dollars for a fifty-pound bag of horse feed is too much."

I always tell them, "You either pay now, or you pay later."

I know I am repeating myself, but this is so important: Paying ahead of time will cost you a lot less, in the long run, than if you have to pay for an emergency. Paying for good health really is an investment because you actually get something out of it: your animals stay healthy.

If you wait until major disease or injury hits, then that treatment becomes a cost, because now you're in the business of fixing. Usually that does not result in a huge improvement in the animal's health. In fact they are often worse than they were before. So it's not an investment; it's a cost.

If, for example, you feed your animal good nutrition all their life, you're investing into their health. But if, let's say, your horse ends up with a colic episode that requires surgery, your animal may get through the colic, but it isn't really any better afterwards; in fact, it is worse because it had to have surgery. Any sort of surgery will affect the body in some way—with scar tissue, for instance—and can cause other problems down the road.

When we do emergency medicine and we wait until something happens, we not only pay more, but we also don't get as much out of that huge amount of money we spent, not to mention the suffering the animal has to go through and the stress and worry we experience.

WHAT DRUGS CAN'T DO FOR YOUR ANIMALS

Do drugs and surgery correct the underlying cause, or do they merely cover up symptoms?

In other words, do you think that animals end up with allergies, for example, because they are lacking prednisolone (a synthetic steroid) in their bodies?

As I explained earlier, there is an underlying cause when an animal is sick, and it is not being addressed by our healthcare system.

Covering Up Symptoms

The conventional healthcare system is very limited in what it can heal. Again, allergies are a perfect example; either you put your animal on prednisone, you use a different shampoo or you give an antihistamine in order to control the symptoms. But as I shared earlier about my own childhood dog, that's what we did. Eventually she ended up with cancer and more health issues. The mainstream conventional medicine really can't heal.

The statistics show that in dogs, for example, 45 percent of dogs over the age of ten will die of cancer. Between 1975 and 1995, the incidence of bladder cancer in dogs examined at veterinary teaching schools in North America increased sixfold.[1] Despite all the research being done, cancer rates continue to climb. When I started veterinary school in 1990, cancer was barely a topic. But today, we hear about cancer every day.

---

[1] Priester W.A., and McKay, F.W. *The occurrence of tumors in domestic animals.* Natl Cancer Inst Monogr 1980; 54:1–210)

Emergent Care Can't Rebuild the Body

The conventional healthcare system is a crisis system, and we have to be aware of that. It works really well for crisis situations. If we have an emergency, we really want to have that system on our side. But it can't really rebuild the body.

For example, if your house is on fire, you want to have firefighters come right away with their axes and water hoses.

But once the fire is extinguished, you don't want to have them come back the next day to help you rebuild the house, right?

That's not what they're for, and that's not what they do. They would do more damage than good. We really need to have someone else come in and rebuild the house. That's really why we need a different healthcare system, and we need a different approach. It's also not helpful to just turn off the fire alarm and ignore the fires that are going on. We need to pay attention to the fire alarm.

The healthcare system is good for emergencies, and that's what you should use it for. If your animal is in a lot of pain, or their quality of life is terrible, then you definitely want to help the animal because it can only heal if it feels better, too. If we really want to rebuild the body, however, we need to rely on a system that focuses on rebuilding health through restoring proper functioning cells.

How Drugs Work

Drugs are in the body for a certain period of time. That's also the time that they are active, and do what they are supposed to do.

But if we don't give the drug the next day, for example, what will happen?

The symptoms will come right back. We have to keep giving the drug over and over again, in order for the symptom to not be present. I say that because, even though you can't see the symptoms, the disease is still going on underneath; the drugs haven't healed anything, really.

I'll use the "check engine" light analogy again: Imagine the "check engine" light comes on and you go to the mechanic to assess what's wrong, but all the mechanic does is reset the light.

What will happen to the car when you drive off?

The light will come right back on.

Wouldn't you be furious if your mechanic did that to you?

That's exactly what the traditional healthcare system does. The drug just resets the light, but it doesn't really fix anything. We have to be aware of that when we treat our animals. Maybe we don't see the symptoms. Maybe the animal is happier and feeling better, but the problem is still there. It hasn't really resolved, and it will continue to fester underneath and come out as something else, and possibly worse than what your animal already has.

We need to really address things in a different way, and also essentially ask why.

Why is the animal sick?

Why is the body not functioning the way it's supposed to?

HOW TO CREATE TRUE HEALING

True healing provides a solution, and a restoration of the body to health. With true healing, the body is repairing whatever is going on. That's what we aim for; we want to restore the body to its optimal function, in order to be able to stop worrying. If we just give drugs and do surgeries, then we still have to continue to worry because things haven't really resolved. True healing has the potential to bring a resolution of the issue that's going on and maximize your animal's health as much as possible.

Holistic Vets and Functional Medicine

As a holistic veterinarian, I investigate the two causes of disease in the attempt to answer why:

- What is interfering with your animal's body?

- What is your animal's body missing?

That's how holistic veterinarians think.

When I work with your animals, I help you provide your animal with what it needs and remove what's interfering with health. One very good example is Wilson, a horse. He had lost a lot of his coat and was really bleached out. Within just a few short weeks of feeding him a good diet, there was a huge difference in the way the animal looked. His coat changed completely within four weeks. It became dark brown, lush, and shiny. There were other things that changed as well, but that was the most noticeable. When you provide the animal's body with what it needs, it can actually do what it's supposed to do.

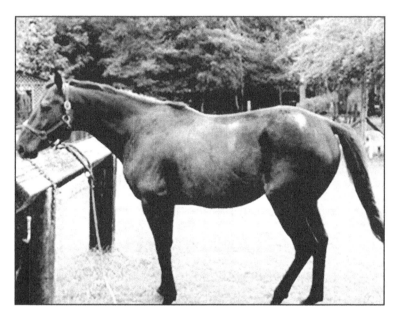

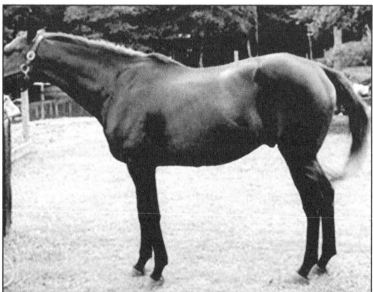

Wilson, before and later, after only 43 days of proper nutrition

When I graduated from veterinary school, my head was filled with all the traditional teachings, but I don't practice most of what I learned. What I practice now is *functional medicine*. Functional medicine is really simple. It's applying natural things to help the body function better.

If you can get your animal's body to function better, what is it going to do?

It's going to improve. When the body heals allergies, for example, at the same time it is healing lack of energy, recurrent infections, pancreatitis, whatever it is that's going on all at the same time. So when the body heals, it heals all at once, and that's because the principles that cause your animal's body to heal are all the same.

Are there any drugs that can do that?

The answer is no.

If you start giving medications to deal with each separate issue, you have to continue to give them. Functional medicine is really an up-and-coming new way of addressing health. It addresses the underlying causes. It asks "why?" It really helps you restore the body to functioning as best as it can.

Doctor Means Teacher

When you try to heal your animals, you need someone to help you. A veterinarian or a doctor is a teacher; *doctor* means *teacher* in Latin. As a veterinarian, it is important that I teach you how to become more independent in caring for your animal's health, so that you don't have to run to the veterinarian all the time. That's really what's lacking in our traditional medical system as well; there is no time for teaching. You go to the vet, they quickly look at the animal, they give you a drug, and then you're out the door and you barely know anything about what's going on. You haven't asked a whole lot of questions, and you haven't been taught a whole lot. We need to change that.

You need to insist that your veterinarian teach you what you need to know. If your veterinarian can't do that, then find another teacher, or read up on the topic. Get as much knowledge as you can, because you are your animal's advocate, and you can't rely on somebody to tell you what to do.

You need to learn and inform yourself, so that you have the knowledge that you need to take care of your animal. You want to be independent. I want you to know what you can do for your animal to keep them healthy to begin with. I want you to be empowered, so that you can also know for yourself, because we're really very similar to our animals.

True healing requires a little bit of work, a little bit of investment, and taking action. Don't just take the battery out of the fire alarm or turn on the vent so that the fire alarm doesn't go off.

Questions and Action Steps

Find a mentor to work with.

The American Holistic Veterinary Medical Association has a list of holistic veterinarians available at www.ahvma.org.

You can also contact me for more information at www.PeakAnimalHealthCenter.com.

CHAPTER FOUR

The Six Pillars to Restore Health

The part can never be well unless the whole is well.
~ Plato

INTRODUCTION TO THE SIX PILLARS

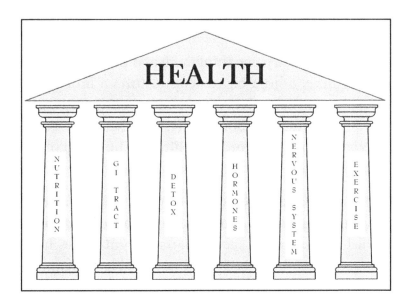

Have you ever tried to improve your animal's health through diet or exercise?

Have you gotten some positive results, only to see your results stall, or maybe even turn in the wrong direction?

Did you ever wonder why, in spite of your best efforts, you didn't achieve your goals and your animal is still suffering?

Simply put, if you do not address the six components of health together, your efforts will most likely fail.

If you only address a portion of the six components of health, you will only get a portion of the results you are expecting to accomplish or no result at all, because all six support and enhance one another.

A lot of people try one thing here and one thing there; for example, a little bit of acupuncture, a little bit of chiropractic, a little bit of herbs, a little bit of this, and a little bit of that, without addressing the whole body. Maybe the animal improves a little bit, but most of the time, the problem remains.

A perfect example is doing chiropractic care on a horse who has gut issues. I can do chiropractic work on it until I'm blue in the face. Unless the gut issues have been addressed, the body will not be able to maintain the adjustments.

By picking and choosing symptoms to treat without addressing the whole system, you're actually wasting a lot of money and precious time. It is likely that your animal will continue to suffer and the underlying problem will continue to cause problems. Your animal could actually get worse. If the animal does get better, maybe their health improves temporarily, but then it will go right back to where it was.

In order to get maximum health for your animal and get it as quickly as possible, you can refer to the Six Pillars. Collectively, they are a systematized way of addressing health concerns. Just as systems are a necessity for any business to be successful, the body needs the same to achieve greater health and well-being.

1. NUTRITION

> *Let food be thy medicine and medicine will be thy food.*
> ~ Hippocrates, 400 BCE

I want to reiterate that a lot of the information on nutrition, especially in the veterinary world, comes from the big companies that make animal food. That goes for dogs, cats, and horses. These big companies have the loudest voices and the biggest marketing budgets. They also infiltrate veterinary schools. They're the ones teaching veterinary students about nutrition.

You can see that there's a conflict of interest there. A lot of the information they promote is based on money, not on what our animals need.

Nutrition Means Life

The MacMillan dictionary states that the definition of food is, "That which is eaten to sustain life, provide energy, promote growth, and repair tissues."

The average diet of dry food, canned food, horse feed, and of course our very own donuts, burgers, fries, and soft drinks do not in any way meet these criteria.

The Standard American Diet (SAD indeed) may provide short-term energy, but it also leads to problems such as:

- Blood sugar imbalance
- Hormone imbalance
- Autoimmune diseases
- Weight gain
- Metabolic diseases
- Cancer

Optimal health must include proper nutrition. Proper diet and clean water are a must. The good news is that it doesn't have to be bland.

Diet is really what sustains our life. It's what provides the cells with the nutrients that they need to be able to function properly. Without the nutrients, the cells can't really do their job, and will end up malfunctioning, which is — as mentioned earlier — disease.

Quality Versus Quantity

The quality of food has declined significantly in the last hundred or so years. Food sources have become deficient. They are exhausted by monoculture. The minerals are bound to the soil when doused with glyphosate (Roundup), making them unavailable to the growing plants.

The quality of food is also largely affected by what ingredients are used. Unfortunately for animal feeds, all the leftovers from the human food industry are added.

For example, in the dog and cat food industry, manufacturers are allowed to include:

- Meat that's no longer fit for human consumption
- Meat from diseased animals
- Old meat
- Euthanized dogs and cats
- Roadkill

The manufacturers can put any number of really disgusting things into dog and cat food that they wouldn't otherwise know what to do with. They're trying to make money off of anything that's available. If they actually had to discard all of it, their expenses would be much higher. They would have to pay to get rid of the waste. It's easier and more profitable to utilize things that otherwise would have to be paid to be thrown away.

Horse food is equally laden with ingredients that promote malfunctioning of cells:

- Wheat middlings
- Soy bean hulls
- Beet pulp (GMO mostly)
- Molasses

Instead of wasting them, pet food manufacturers are trying to make a buck on it by putting these ingredients into horse food. Unfortunately, what gets into these feeds is largely damaging to the animal's health, and in no way promotes health.

Food either heals or harms, and most commercially available foods harm.

Pottenger's Cats

There is one very important study that was done in the 1940s by Dr. Francis M. Pottenger. He was a medical doctor doing a study with humans who had tuberculosis. He was using cat adrenal gland extract to support these patients, to see if he could make them feel better. When people heard about his study, they started dumping cats on his doorstep. He ended up with nine hundred cats. Because he couldn't feed them all raw food from the butcher's he had to feed some of them a cooked diet. Soon he started noticing that there was a difference in health between the cats who ate raw food and the cats who ate cooked food.

Pottenger decided to do a study.

He separated the cats into two groups: one group ate a raw-only diet.

The other group was getting a mix of about two-thirds cooked meat and one-third raw milk.

Because he wanted to see the effects on future generations, his study continued through four generations of cats.

The cats on the raw food diet remained healthy for four generations. Nothing changed; one generation after another, they stayed healthy while eating the raw food diet.

The ones on the cooked-food and milk diet developed degenerative diseases and became lazy towards the end of life within the first generation. In the second generation, they developed degenerative diseases and illnesses in the middle of life and had some loss of coordination. In the third generation, they developed diseases and illnesses in the beginning of life, and many died before six months of age.

There were many problems in the third generation:

- Blindness and weakness from birth
- Reproductive issues
- Parasites
- Skin diseases
- Allergies
- Soft, pliable bones
- Adverse personality changes

The fourth generation was not even produced: the third generation parents were either sterile, or the fourth generation cats were aborted before birth. In other words, there was no fourth generation produced.

We have to take into consideration that in the 1940s, any cooked food was likely of much higher quality than any cooked or processed cat food that we can get today. It would be difficult to do this sort of multigenerational study currently, because we render our animals sterile by neutering and spaying them. We can't really see how health would continue, and whether the cats could reproduce. But overall, health has been declining, and younger animals are getting sick with diseases that used to be seen in older individuals only (Cushing's disease in horses used to occur almost exclusively in old mares).

Other ailments affecting the Pottenger cats included:

- Respiratory issues
- Gastrointestinal issues
- Constitutional problems and disorders
- Hypothyroidism
- Inflammation
- Dental malocclusions

Dental malocclusions occurred because the cats were starting to lose some of the bone structure in the head. So, some of the third-generation cats were actually missing part of the facial bones, or the bones of the head and skull.

Dr. Price—who was a dentist in the same era—was studying indigenous people. Compared to our western civilization, these people who were eating natural foods found in their environment had exceptionally good dental alignment. Most of our children today need to have braces because their teeth are so misaligned. There is definitely a parallel between Dr. Pottenger's observation and Dr. Price's.

Then he also wanted to find out how long it would take to regenerate these cats; to see how long it would take for them to return to optimum health.

He returned first- and second-generation cooked-meat-fed cats to a raw diet. Their offspring were maintained on a raw diet as well. He found that it takes about four generations to regenerate to normal health. In the second generation, there was some improvement in resistance to disease. In the third generation, allergies were persisting, and skeletal and soft tissue changes were still noticeable, but to a lesser degree. In the fourth generation, most of the deficiency signs and symptoms disappeared, but seldom completely. Based on that, we can see that by not feeding a species-appropriate diet, we are really doing damage.

Dr. Pottenger also tested the value of cat excreta as fertilizer. He found that plants would not grow in the presence of waste from cats that ate cooked food. Even the plants don't really like that.

Species-Appropriate Diet

As an example of what good nutrition does, let's look at cell membranes. Cell membranes are a little bit like a switch station in old-fashioned telephone connections. For those who are too young, when somebody wanted to make a call, they'd pick up the phone and an operator would answer. You'd tell the operator the number of the person you wanted to speak to, and the operator would physically connect your line or wire to a port to that other person's wire.

That's the function of cell membranes. Cell membranes are the connectors between the outside of the cell and the inside of the cell. There are a lot of nutrients that float around and want to get into a cell. The cell membranes control the flow into and out of the cells. It's very important that cell membranes work well.

Another way to think of the cell membrane is that it is like your skin. You don't want things to go into your body that aren't supposed to, and you don't want to have things pour out of your body that shouldn't. Cell membranes are a bit like that.

Cell membranes are dependent on good fats, good protein, and also some carbohydrates. It is really important that you nourish your animal's body so that these cell membranes can do their job.

If they break, two results can occur:

1. The cell membrane leaks. The inside of the cell goes outside the cell, causing damage and inflammation. At the same time, too much gets into the cell.

2. The cell membrane becomes *impermeable*. The cell can neither absorb nutrients, nor excrete waste. The cell dies from a buildup of toxins and lack of nourishment.

Becky is a perfect example of how simply optimizing nutrition can turn things around. She is a middle-aged mare with chronically sore hooves. Ever since I met her she has moved very stiffly. After changing her nutrition to an anti-inflammatory diet, the soreness disappeared and so did some of the extra pounds she was carrying around.

The Price We Pay for Poor Nutrition

I know that buying good nutrition for your animal can be costly, but if you don't give them good nutrition they can end up with toxicities and deficiencies, which then cause the cells to malfunction. Feeding cheap feed with low-quality ingredients that are harmful to the body will end up in high vet bills, layups, and emotional distress among other discomforts. The price that you pay for poor nutrition is really high, not just financially, but obviously your animal will not be feeling as well and enjoy its life as much as it could. Plus, any time your animals are sick, you also feel sick.

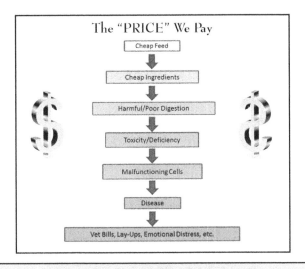

The "PRICE" We Pay

Cheap Feed → Cheap Ingredients → Harmful/Poor Digestion → Toxicity/Deficiency → Malfunctioning Cells → Disease → Vet Bills, Lay-Ups, Emotional Distress, etc.

Questions and Action Steps:

How much are you spending per month on food and supplements for your animals?

How much are you spending on veterinary care?

What are you feeding your animals?

What are the ingredients?

Learn how to read and interpret a label.

Take a trip to a natural pet store and talk to the owner about a species-appropriate diet.

Ask if they have samples.

Use filtered water for your animals.

2. GI TRACT: NO GUT, NO GLORY

All diseases begin in the gut.
~ Hippocrates, 400 BCE

Many diseases that seem to be totally unrelated to the gut–such as back pain, skin issues, or arthritis to just name a few–are actually caused by gastro-intestinal disturbances. The gut is connected to everything that happens in the whole body.

Diseases that are linked to poor GI function include:

Diseases Linked to Leaky Gut	
• Anemia	• Itchy skin rash
• Hypoglycemia	• Seborrhea
• Elevated liver enzymes	• Thin hair
• Low white blood cell count	• Lymphadenopathy
• Mineral deficiency	• Hypokalemic periodic paralysis
• Appetite ↑ or ↓	• Founder/Laminitis
• Loss of vitality	• Muscle wasting
• Cardiac issues	• Muscle weakness
• Abdominal distension and pain	• Epilepsy
• GI ulcers	• Peripheral neuropathy
• Diarrhea, constipation	• Tremors
• Irritable bowel disease	• Vasculitis of the central nervous system
• Defective tooth enamel	• Pneumonia
• Vomiting	• Cataracts
• Malabsorption	• Dry eye
• Small intestinal bacterial overgrowth	• Uveitis
• Addison's disease (adrenal fatigue)	• Arthritis
	• Kidney stones

• Cushing's disease	• Urinary tract infection (UTI)
• Hepatitis	• Infertility
• Autoimmune thyroiditis	• Miscarriage
• Diabetes mellitus type I	• Complications during
• Pancreatic insufficiency	pregnancy, labor, and
• Allergies	delivery
• Asthma	• Failure to thrive
• Immunodeficiency	• Hyperactivity
• Food sensitivities	• Restlessness
• IgA deficiency	• Timid behavior
• Systemic lupus	• Anxiety
erythematosus	• Depression
• Urticaria (hives)	• Aggression
• Hair loss	• Dementia
• Eczema	• Reduced learning
• Edema (swelling)	

For us humans, the list also includes:	
• Acne	• Osteoporosis
• Chronic fatigue	• Migraine
• Fibromyalgia	• Alzheimer's
• Autism	• Psoriasis
• Parkinson's	

The Importance of the GI Tract

You can see that there are a lot of diseases that are linked to the gut. Just like with everything else in the body, the gut really hasn't changed, as far as its ability to digest things, such as, for example, carbohydrates in dogs and cats. Their GI tract is not made for that. They, in fact, don't have the enzymes to digest carbohydrates. We need to feed the gut what it can deal with, and not create an imbalance. The same is true with horses. If we feed too much grain, too many easily digestible starches, we create an acidosis in the hindgut, which causes ulcerations and damage to the gut lining.

Leaky Gut and Its Effects on the Entire System

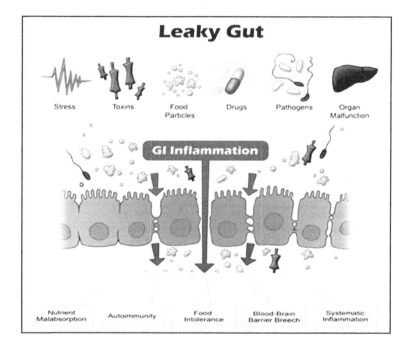

The gut lining or epithelium is made of a single layer of cells and adjacent to that are blood vessels. There is a very close connection between the food that comes down the esophagus and the blood. There's only the epithelium that separates the digesta from the blood. It is responsible for digesting the food and processing it so that nutrients can be absorbed into the bloodstream and used by the body.

In a normal, healthy gut, the individual cells are very closely tied together through tight junctions, so that nothing can pass between the cells and go directly into the bloodstream. Little finger-like structures at the lumen side of the cell contain enzymes and host the microbes that help with digestion. In a healthy gut, anything that is ingested is broken down, absorbed into the cells, and then transported into the bloodstream.

In an inflamed gut, these little tight junctions that are connecting the individual cells and keeping them really close together break down. As they break down, particles can pass between cells that have not been properly digested and are too big for the body to use.

As these particles get into the bloodstream, the immune system has to clean them up, because they are not supposed to be there. The body recognizes them as foreign bodies and sends the immune system to clean up.

Any time the immune system comes running, guess what's happening?

We have inflammation, because that's what the immune system does. It creates inflammation to clean up, to heal, and then, theoretically — in a normal case — the inflammation will subside once the threat is over.

With a leaky gut, this threat is never over; it continues to stimulate the immune system, which then causes inflammation body-wide. Because the particles that go directly into the bloodstream cannot be used by the body, nutritional deficiency develops. Even though the food goes into the body, it's not in a form the cells can use.

Another problem with this leaky gut is the development of food sensitivities. If a protein particle, chicken for example, enters the bloodstream not fully digested, the body starts to have a reaction to the chicken.

So any time the dog or cat will eat the chicken, the immune system says, "Wait a minute, that's the one that was causing problems; let me attack it."

This perpetuates inflammation in the GI tract, because now it has become sensitive to chicken. That's how nutritional sensitivities develop, resulting in symptoms like chronic ear infections, skin allergies, hot spots, hives, and more.

Any time inflammation is present in the gut, there is also inflammation created in the brain. The gut and brain are very closely related. The chemicals produced during the inflammatory process affect the blood-brain barrier, which normally keeps things out of the brain that aren't supposed to be there. The chemicals basically cause the barrier to leak. Chemicals enter the brain, causing imbalances that can result in behavioral issues, for example. Over time, the imbalance destroys neurons, which then can result in dementia.

Do you remember the progression of health issues in my childhood dog, Windy?

Inflammation in the GI tract will also affect the liver, for example, because it is in close proximity to the GI tract and inflammation tends to move back up into the liver via the bile duct. The same is true for the pancreas, which is also connected to the intestines through a small duct. It too can respond to inflammation in the GI tract and become destroyed over time.

The triggers causing intestinal damage can be:

- Dietary protein
- Low HCL (stomach acid)
- Low enzymes
- Antibiotics
- Infections
- Blood sugar issues

- Stress
- Toxins
- Hormone imbalances
- Food allergies

Helpful Helpers: Gut Microbes

Unless you've lived a life devoid of modern communication devices, research of the connection between microbes and health has been hard to miss. Just about any ailment plaguing humanity is being looked at from a microbial angle.

The microbiome is the entirety of microbes that share our body space. These microbes are generally nonpathogenic and exist in harmony and symbiotically with their host. Symbiosis means that the microbes and the body mutually benefit from one another. Trillions of microbes are part of the human body. Microbes outnumber human cells by a factor of ten. In other words, we're mostly microbes.

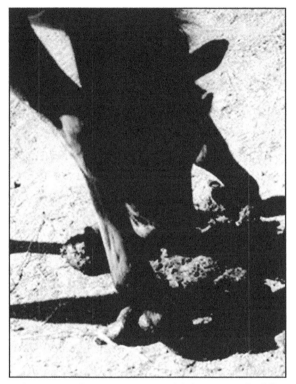

Foal ingesting fecal matter to establish its microbial flora

Initial exposure to microbes comes from the birth canal. Animals will also commonly replenish their digestive flora by eating feces. As disgusting as this sounds, "eating shit" promotes a healthy life.

Daisy, a very proper poodle lady used to be very picky about the poop she would choose. On our walks she paid no attention to some horse manure piles, while others seemed to be a delicacy.

Foals often eat their mother's feces as they transition to eating more solid food. Horses with GI issues can also at times be found dining on their pasture mates' excrement to heal their gut.

In the wild, dogs and cats tend to first feast on the intestines of their prey, thereby ingesting large amounts of microorganisms. Dogs will also much enjoy a buffet of rotting meat and further increase the intake of microbes.

The microbiome plays a MAJOR role in physical and mental health:

- Intestinal maturation
- Inhibition of pathogen growth
- Digestion of food
- Protection of mucosal barrier (prevention of leaky gut)
- Regulation of hormones
- Excretion of toxins
- Production of vitamins and other healing compounds
- Training the immune system and modulating immune response
- Production of secretory IgA (immune globulins)
- Neural development
- Synthesis of neurotransmitters (90 percent of serotonin is made in the GI tract)

With 80 percent of the body's immune system residing in the gastrointestinal tract, we can easily deduce that its health is paramount to the proper functioning of the entire body.

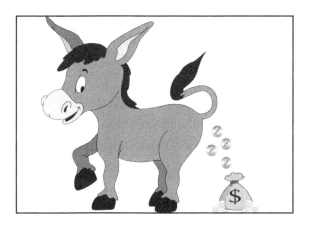

Microbiome research is one of the hottest fields of study and yields information about a most promising treatment. Likely it will revolutionize medicine and how we treat disease. In humans the microbiome is found to play a role in diseases like:

- Diabetes
- Rheumatoid arthritis
- MS
- Fibromyalgia
- Allergies
- Obesity
- Anxiety and depression
- Some cancers

Since microbes in the gut play an important role in the production of neurotransmitters, a disturbance in gut flora affects the brain, potentially causing psychological disorders such as depression, schizophrenia, anxiety, and other neurochemical imbalances.

A few veterinarians including Dr. Margo Romano and I are successfully using Microbiome Restorative Therapy (MBRT) in our practices. MBRT is the practice of transferring fecal matter from a healthy individual's intestines into those of a sick individual. The process of transplantation is very simple. Finding a healthy fecal donor on the other hand can be tricky. Many criteria need to be met in order for this process to work. The donor must be in excellent health and also be free of chemical exposure. The recipient's gut has to be prepared for a transplant to give the newly introduced biome a chance to survive and thrive.

Symptoms and diseases that can benefit from MBRT include:

- Gastro-intestinal disturbances
- Neurological issues
- Hypothyroidism
- Aggression
- Anxiety
- Skin conditions
- Cancers

- Lyme disease
- Kidney and liver issues
- Chronic ear infections

I've seen some incredible changes in many of the animals I've given "shit," so to speak. Bear, a German shepherd with longstanding IBD (inflammatory bowel disease) had normal feces within just a few days after receiving his transplant. His anxiety level decreased tremendously and all he wanted to do was play.

Maisy, an elderly Jack Russell lady with considerable skin allergies, slept for two days after her treatment. She was probably exhausted from all the scratching. She then perked up full of energy and her itchiness was significantly reduced.

Chief is a horse whose greatest weakness was his GI tract. He had a severe case of leaky gut.

> *I had a twelve-year-old gelding who couldn't be ridden because he was unpredictable. Many vets examined him in hopes of determining what was creating such extreme behavior. But after several years and countless suggestions, I gave up. Dr. Suter did for my gelding what I thought was impossible: she transformed him from a pasture ornament to a wonderful, giving, trusted partner.*
>
> ~ Misty N.

Treatments

Healing the gastrointestinal tract is paramount if you want a healthy animal. If your animal can't properly process the food it eats, the body will become deficient. If the gut lining is leaking, the body will be invaded with food particles and microbes. The resulting inflammation will prevent healing and actually continue to fuel disease.

So, what does it take to heal your animal's gut?

The Institute for Functional Medicine has come up with the *Four R Program*:

1. Remove: Undertake an elimination diet.

- Remove the common allergy-producing foods and processed foods.

- Treat chronic infections (yeast, unhealthy bacteria, parasites).

2. Replace: Investigate digestive aids.

- Use digestive herbs, digestive enzymes, or other digestive supports that can help protect the lining from further damage, and coat the intestines while they heal.

- Provide healthy diet.

3. Reinoculate: Rebalance gut flora

- Give probiotics to re-introduce proper flora to intestines.

- Get a fecal transplant for your animal.

4. Repair: Rebuild your animal's intestinal cells

- Add amino acids such as L-glutamine, pantothenic acid, zinc, omega-3 EPA/fish oil, vitamin E, amino acid glycine, into your animal's diet.

Questions and Action Steps

Eliminate high carbohydrate and processed foods and replace them with species-appropriate diet:

- Read labels.

- Provide probiotics.

- Add enzymes.

- Give omega-3s (animal-based for carnivores and plant-based for herbivores).

---

3. DETOXIFICATION

*The best way to detoxify
is to stop putting toxic things into the body.*
~ Andrew Weil

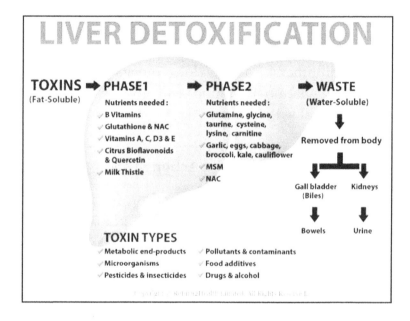

Toxic Exposure

Our animals' bodies are designed to take in nutrition, use what they can, and get rid of what is not useful. All of our animals' cells produce waste, and this waste needs to be removed. The liver is one of the main organs for detoxification.

Toxins get into the liver where they are transformed in a couple of steps into waste products that can be excreted either by the gall bladder and feces, or by the kidney and urine. In order for the liver to be able to do its job, it needs nutrients for both of these steps.

Again, there is a connection to good nutrition that you need to provide the liver in order for it to do its job.

Now, if the liver does not have nutrients, or the liver is overloaded with toxins, it will not be able to function as well as it could. Toxins will get backlogged in the body and cause inflammation. The liver was made to deal with an amount of toxicity that is much less than typical levels today. You have to compare toxicity yesterday with how it is today.

Remember that more than 1.5 million new chemicals have been put on the market since World War II? Most of them are carcinogenic and have never been tested for safety. Eighty thousand of those interfere with hormones. They're called xenoestrogens, meaning that they mimic estrogen, and as such, they act as endocrine disrupters.

Estrogen is highly inflammatory and causes a lot of issues, such as:

- Cancer
- Infertility
- Metabolic diseases

Girls, for example, are developing breast tissue and having their periods much earlier in life, because of these xenoestrogens. They are very damaging to the body. They create inflammation and hormonal imbalance.

As mentioned earlier, in the 1920s, fewer than one million pounds of chemicals were produced in the United States. In the year 2000, up to 140 plus *billion* pounds of synthetic chemicals produced per year. That's an incredible increase.

Do you think that the body is able to tolerate this onslaught of toxins and can deal with it?

I would say no, the body has not evolved to be able to handle that amount of toxicity. You need to help the body detoxify on a regular basis, so that it can continue to function somewhat properly. If you don't do that, your animal friend ends up with toxin accumulation, and failure of health down the road.

Where do these toxins all come from?

As discussed in Chapter Two, there are many, many sources.

In the water supply, for example, you can find:

- Chlorine
- Fluoride

- Pharmaceutical drug residues
- Pesticides
- Herbicides
- Fertilizers

In the food supply, there may be:

- Artificial sweeteners like high fructose corn syrup
- Preservatives
- Food components sourced from contaminated areas
- Poor quality ingredients
- Car exhaust
- Industrial air pollutants
- Drugs
- Genetically modified organisms (GMOs) in corn and soy

Those are just a few of the ways in which your animals may be exposed to toxins. The body can become toxic to itself. If your animals have an accumulation of toxins in the body and an increase of chronic inflammation, this chronic inflammation will produce chemicals in the body that are toxic to the cells. These chemicals are good for acute cases; for example, if your animal friend hits his leg on something, the body needs inflammation to heal the bruised area. But if there is ongoing inflammation, these same chemicals keep being produced and become damaging to the body. It then becomes a vicious cycle and the body will become more and more toxic as it goes on.

If we don't detoxify, our animals are bound to get sick down the road, or at the very least not feel as well as they could; it's pretty much a guarantee.

Questions and Action Steps:

Go through your house and read the labels of the cleaning products you regularly use:

- Laundry detergent
- All soap products
- Shampoos
- Toilet cleaners
- Window cleaners

Do you know what the ingredients are?

Can you pronounce them?

My philosophy is that if I don't know what a chemical is, I don't buy or use it. Try to find safer alternatives. Check all of the products you use on the Environmental Working Group website (EWG. org) to find out if they're safe.

Are you remodeling your house or getting new furniture or carpeting?

New products tend to outgas toxins and may become a problem for you, your families, and your animals.

Observe your neighbors to be aware when they might be spraying toxic chemicals on their lawns, gardens, or orchards. Keep your animals inside during this time. Wash their paws with a little bit of hypoallergenic soap to remove chemicals after exposure.

4. HORMONES

When endocrine patterns change,
it alters the way you think and feel.
One shift in the pattern tends to trip another.
~ Hilary Mantel

Hilary Mantel said it well. We women know all about that — don't we?

All the organs and glands in our body serve very important purposes, within the overall function of the body.

Hormone glands are essential to maintain health, such as:

- Maintenance of healthy weight
- Healthy body structure
- Energy production
- Behavior and mood
- Proper metabolism
- Digestion

Hormone glands include:

- Adrenals
- Ovaries
- Testes
- Pancreas
- Thyroid

These glands produce the hormones that send chemical messages to communicate within the body. There are hundreds of different hormones within the body that work daily to make your animal's body a well-oiled machine, and regulate everything in their bodies.

Hormones in General

A small abnormality or imbalance in the endocrine system will throw off the regulatory balance and affect the way cells function.

Causes of hormonal imbalances can be:

- Poor diet
- Sedentary lifestyle
- Stress
- Pain
- Behavior
- Body composition and structural issues
- Toxicity (internal and external)

The imbalance or decline can occur rapidly or slowly over the years. If hormones are not properly evaluated or brought into balance, optimal health is not obtainable. Too often, hormones and the endocrine system don't receive any attention.

The Thyroid Hormone

The thyroid gland is one of the master hormone glands that affects everything. The thyroid gland is located in the throat area, in proximity of the Adam's apple in humans, and animals as well.

The thyroid gland produces two different hormones: One is T4 and one is T3. T4 is the inactive form and is produced in the greatest amount: 80 to 90 percent. T3 is the active thyroid hormone, and that is present in about 10 to 20 percent. Just like crude oil has to be transformed into gasoline, T4 has to be changed into T3. T3 in this example would be like gasoline. The body really needs the gasoline in order to run and to function. T4 is basically the reserve, so that the body can convert it into T3 if more is needed.

Can you guess where the majority of this conversion takes place?

In the liver!

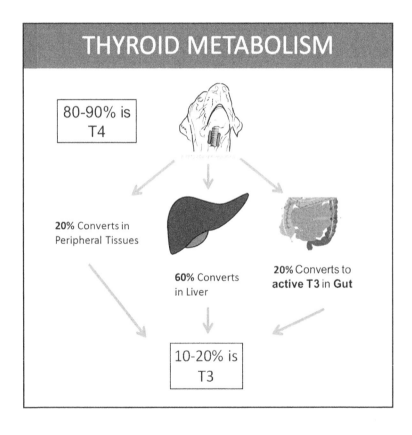

You can see that the thyroid gland is very much dependent on the liver functioning properly, but the liver is also dependent on the thyroid hormone. They can't work without each other, and because the liver needs good nutrition in order to function well, we have a connection to good diet here, as well.

The thyroid, of course, also needs nutrients like iodine in order to produce the thyroid hormones. If the animal does not have enough iodine in their diet, they may not be able to produce enough from the T3 and T4 hormones.

A caveat about testing: when your veterinarian tests your animal's thyroid, usually they test T4 only; they don't test T3, or any other parameters of the thyroid hormone. That is troublesome, because as you probably realize now, if we only measure T4, we don't know how much of that T4 is actually being activated into T3 in the liver, in the gut, or other tissues. Measuring T4 just tells us how much crude oil we have, but we don't know how much of that crude oil has been transformed into gasoline.

The thyroid hormone is really important for every cell. Without the thyroid hormone, the cells cannot do their jobs. That's like trying to drive a car without gasoline; nothing will happen.

Or, if you put a cake batter in the oven at 100°F, what will happen?

Not much. There's not going to be a cake. The same is true for the body. We need enough thyroid hormone for all of the processes to run at the right speed and the right temperature.

Testing

I mentioned testing of the thyroid gland, but there are other hormones that can be tested for as well, such as estrogen, for example. When we test hormone levels, it's really important that we get an overall view of what's going on with the hormonal system, because hormones interact with each other. If one is out of balance, another one will become out of balance, as well. For example, progesterone and estrogen need to be in balance.

Testing is important because we need to know what is going on. If your animal's thyroid isn't functioning as well as it should, a number of symptoms will develop that can only be fixed by restoring proper thyroid function.

Spaying and Neutering

It is commonplace to remove vital organs such as the ovaries and testicles. These organs are essential for maintenance of health such as a healthy weight and body structure for example.

Recently, the side effects of spaying and neutering have gained more attention.

Several studies have found significant health risks related to spaying and neutering:

- Increased risk for cardiac tumors and bone cancer
- Abnormal bone growth and development
- Higher rate of cranial cruciate ligament ruptures in dogs
- Hip dysplasia
- Lymphangiosarcoma
- Lymphosarcoma mast cell tumors
- Urinary incontinence
- Hypothyroidism
- Infectious diseases
- Adverse reactions to vaccines
- Increased behavioral problems

Our animals really need all of their hormones in order for their body to function properly.

One of my patients is a two-year-old, mixed-breed dog who started gaining weight after she was spayed. Her hormones became so deregulated that her weight doubled. There had been no change in the amount of food she was receiving. Her thyroid hormone levels had dropped so low that she became morbidly obese at that young age. Thankfully, providing her with bio-identical hormone replacement turned her health around and she became an energetic, playful young dog.

Spaying and neutering are common practices, but they do have consequences—sometimes severe consequences. Thankfully there are alternatives that prevent reproduction without removing these vitally important glands.

For alternatives, see my website at www.PeakAnimalHealthCenter.com.

Questions and Action Steps:

Is your animal behaving appropriately?

Is your animal vibrant?

Get their thyroid tested. Ask for a full thyroid panel (Lab info on www.PeakAnimalHealthCenter.com).

For horses: test their morning temperature with a glass thermometer (before 9 a.m. and before eating if possible). Their temperature should be between 100°F and 100.8°F.

If it is below 99.6°F, your horse is likely to be showing symptoms such as:

- Low energy
- Recurrent thrush
- Slow shedding
- Insulin resistance
- Weight gain
- Poor topline
- Chronic GI issues

If you're a responsible guardian, reconsider the need for spaying and neutering.

Avoid estrogenic compounds and other endocrine disruptors (for more info, see www. PeakAnimalHealthCenter.com).

---

5. NERVOUS SYSTEM

Anything's possible if you've got enough nerve.
~ J. K. Rowling

The nervous system is like a conduit or a phone line. It gets information from the external and internal environment.

Examples of the external environment are:

- Precipitation
- Temperature
- Wind
- Touch

The internal environment includes:

- Skin
- Muscles
- Teeth
- GI tract
- Heart
- Liver
- Lungs

It also receives feedback from emotions and from memory (whatever your animal's experience of life has been).

The central nervous system (brain and spinal cord) processes all of that information and sends feedback to the body to tell it what to do.

One way this happens is through muscle response; moving, for example. So if there were an emotion of fear in a horse, their muscles would be activated in order to be able to run away from the threat.

The other output system is the autonomic response.

The autonomic nervous system is that part of the nervous system that we don't have conscious control over, such as:

- Peristalsis in the GI tract
- Heart rate
- Blood pressure

In the example of the scared horse, heart rate would increase and blood vessels to the muscles would dilate to supply them with more oxygen.

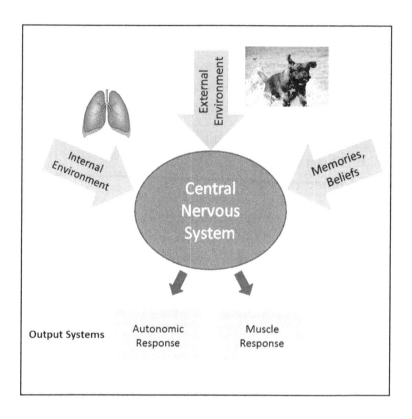

There are hundreds of chemicals called neurotransmitters that are part of the nervous system. They connect and transmit signals from one nerve to another.

Examples of neurotransmitters are:

- Serotonin
- Melatonin
- Acetylcholine
- Adrenalin

- Dopamine
- Endorphins

This ties us back into nutrition, doesn't it?

Good nutrition is crucial to make all of these neurotransmitters that allow the nervous system to run smoothly.

Poor Nerve Transmission

One area where the nervous system commonly gets affected is in the space where the nerves exit the spinal cord, which is between two adjacent vertebrae. This space is called the *intervertebral foramen*. When the spine becomes misaligned due to uneven tension of the muscles around the spine, the little joints (facet joints) connecting the vertebrae become inflamed. As a result, the nerve exit space narrows and compresses the blood supply to the nerves. Decreased amounts of oxygen to the nerve then limit transmission of nerve signals to the tissues they innervate. This affects how an animal is able to move and how quickly it can respond to a stimulus.

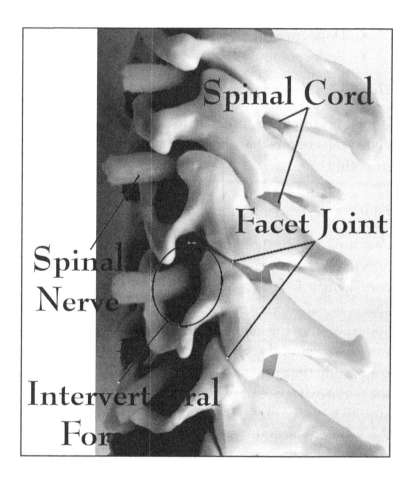

For example, let's say, your horse is inadvertently stepping into a hole. The muscles are supposed to respond quickly to the incoming information (the stimulus that there's uneven ground underfoot) to avoid damage to the leg. But if nerve conduction is slow, this won't happen and they may tear a tendon or ligament.

Internal organs are affected as well.

Impaired nerve transmission can interrupt normal function and create conditions, such as:

- Urinary incontinence
- Constipation
- Heart palpitations

Can you see how important it is that your animal doesn't have any kinks in these communication lines?

When one area of the body is affected it will cause a series of compensations and affect other areas as a result. I see this especially in horses with GI issues; they usually have back pain. That's because the nerves from the GI tract enter the spinal cord at the same levels as those coming from the back muscles. If the nerves from the GI tract are irritated, they will irritate other nerves around them. As a result, the nerves coming from the back muscles send irritated information to the brain as well, which the brain will interpret as pain. If I were to just address the back pain, the horse might feel a little bit better for a couple of days, but the soreness would come right back because the underlying cause had not been addressed.

It is so important that you understand that trying to eliminate a symptom (in this case, back pain) doesn't fix the problem (GI issues).

Healing the Nervous System

One particular way you can assure that the nervous system of your animal friend is functioning properly is through bodywork. Chiropractic care is one of the best modalities for that, but there are others such as osteopathy and cranio-sacral therapy.

The goal is to restore proper range of motion in the spinal joints, but also in other joints in order to reestablish good nerve transmission.

What happens if you do nothing to maintain your car? Let's say you don't do any oil changes. That's like ignoring the fact that your animal also needs maintenance work to preserve proper motion of joints. If nothing is done they often end up with joint degeneration in certain areas, which in the long run causes arthritis.

You may not see the arthritic changes tomorrow, but maybe in a few years your dog will have a hard time getting up or your horse will have degenerative hock changes and be lame.

When your vet finds arthritic changes on radiographs, it means some form of imbalance is present. Arthritis is really like an archeological finding; meaning that it simply indicates something has been going on for a long time. The body has been compensating and has built up more bone, trying to make up for the weakness and create more stability. That didn't happen overnight.

So, why not prevent these issues from happening?

Once the damage has been done, a common strategy in conventional veterinary medicine is to inject joints with anti-inflammatory drugs or use medication to manage related pain. If we find the imbalances and weaknesses and fix them as they occur rather than wait for things to go wrong, we could avoid the high cost and side effects from these treatments. Not to mention we could spare our animals years of discomfort.

With proper preventative care (regular chiropractic adjustments, for example) you can prevent a lot of issues down the road. I myself see a chiropractor once a month to maintain proper alignment and joint and organ health in my body.

Aside from keeping the musculoskeletal system working like a well-oiled machine, your animal's body will also be more resistant to disease, have better organ function and just feel good overall.

The nervous system is like a computer. We want it to run smoothly, we want it to be fast, and we don't want it to get stuck or shut down. We want to make sure that the nervous system is fully functioning and there are no interruptions in the lines of communication.

Quito (the horse I mentioned earlier who had GI irritation that caused his grumpiness) had damaged a tendon in his front leg. Upon examination I noticed that he had tremendous tightness as well as pain in his lower neck.

Now, you might ask what his tight neck has to do with his tendon injury. The base of the neck is where the nerves innervating the muscle that is connected to the damaged tendon exit the spine.

Quito's nerves weren't able to innervate the muscle properly and the muscle became weak. Any time a muscle is weak, the tendons and ligaments have to pick up the slack. But they're not made for that. If there is chronic tension on tendons and ligaments, they can become damaged either chronically or acutely.

In Quito's case we can take our inquiry a step further.

What caused tightness in his neck in the first place?

You guessed right! His irritated GI tract created compensatory tightness in many areas of his body, including his neck. Everything is connected.

Another example of long-term imbalance can be seen in cruciate ligament tears in dogs. The cruciate ligaments' job is to stabilize the femur and the tibia, because they're aligned at an angle. The cruciate ligaments are supposed to hold them together, but the muscles across the joint play an even bigger role in the stabilization of the knee joint as well. If these muscles become weak, then there's extra tension on the cruciate ligaments. They have to take up the slack, which can result in little micro-tears, and eventually a complete tear, if it comes to it. The issue usually originates in the pelvic (lumbo-sacral) area, because that's where the sciatic nerve exits the spinal cord.

The sciatic nerve innervates the majority of the hind leg muscles and is thus very important. It tends to get compressed under the piriformis muscle, which is a small muscle that you might have felt if you've ever had a massage and somebody dug their elbow into our butt. It's the one that can be really painful under pressure. The piriformis muscle puts tension on the sciatic nerve if there's a misalignment in the pelvic area such as torsion.

Any issue with the sciatic nerve results in weakness of many muscles along the hind leg. The joints become unstable. In dogs, most of that manifests as instability in the knee, which then can result in tears.

Spaying and neutering can perpetuate this instability, especially when done at a time when the animal is still growing. In spayed and neutered animals, bones continue to grow longer than they should because important regulatory input is missing. The growth plates of the tibia and femur close at different times in the development and removing sex hormones alters this process, resulting in a straighter hind leg that is more prone to injuries.

Dog Collars, Injuries, and Stress

Dog collars are a big problem, because if a dog lunges on a leash while wearing one, that extra force on the neck can cause major problems to the nervous system. It's a bit like getting whiplash every time they pull or jerk on the leash. If they're running at full speed and all of the sudden they hit the end of the leash, it can cause a big problem. I see a lot of neck issues as a result.

There's some question about whether dog collars affect the thyroid gland, also located in the neck. If you constantly put pressure on that thyroid gland, which is really quite superficial, right under the skin, the damage to that thyroid gland could affect the hormones at some point, too.

All the nerves that go to the body have to go through the cervical spine. Stress to the neck is therefore a big problem, because it will affect every single nerve and the entire body. Pronged collars dig in around the neck and that's especially problematic.

Obviously, if your dog never pulls on its collar, that's a different story. Alternatively, a harness is a much better choice because it puts a little bit of pressure in different areas and they don't have that same jerking effect on the neck. That's something to consider.

Of course when it comes to restraining your animal the primary goal is to keep your animal and yourself safe.

Questions and Action Steps

Get regular bodywork for your animal (see www. PeakAnimalHealthCenter.com for resources).

Get a harness for your dog if possible.

Use an equine dentist who specializes in balancing your horse's mouth properly (see the Teeth section in the appendix).

Learn more about your horse's hooves and what they should look like (see www. PeakAnimalHealthCenter.com).

Can you hear your dog's toenails tapping the floor as they walk?

Trim your dog's nails regularly. They should not touch the ground. You should not be able to hear them when they walk on a hard surface (see www. PeakAnimalHealthCenter.com).

> *I did get a chance to work Ellie (horse) yesterday and she is MUCH better, back to her normal gait! That pinched nerve must have really bothered her. Glad we got it taken care of before I left town again. Thank you!*
>
> ~ Lori K.

Emma is a dachshund who had back surgery several years ago. Although no longer paralyzed, she still suffers from the degenerative changes that ensued. Here is her guardian's experience:

> *Dr. Suter performed a simple canine neurological exam consisting of manually curling Emma's back paws and waiting for Emma's response. Emma simply stood, paws still curled, with no intention, awareness, nor strength to uncurl them. Dr. Suter proceeded to work on her through chiropractic medicine and tried the test once more. Not only did Emma immediately right her paws, but she took off, chasing a nearby dog, running with power, speed, and as straight as an arrow! Tears came to my eyes . . . .*
>
> ~ Aly S.

6. FITNESS AND EXERCISE

Fit is not a destination, it's a way of life.
~ Author unknown

Animals are not made to be couch potatoes or stuck in a dark stall somewhere. Animals are made to move. Obviously, different species have different requirements. Dogs and cats, for example tend to sleep many, many hours a day, whereas horses sleep very little and stand and move constantly. In order to get the best health possible for your animal, you need to imitate what natural demands for movement would be.

For a horse that would mean moving around pretty much twenty-four hours a day, seven days a week. It does not have to be at high speed, just moving around and walking several miles. Wild horses are known to travel up to thirty miles per day. We have to make it possible for animals to move the way they would in nature. For dogs and cats, exercise is mostly from walking around to see if they can find some prey somewhere, and if they do see prey somewhere, then they pick up speed and have to really exert themselves to hunt. It's important that we work with their physiology.

The Benefits of Movement

The benefits are multiple. For one, it keeps blood circulation going. Good blood flow is important for all cells to get their nutrients, and to be able to get rid of waste. It helps with balancing hormones, because if your animal exercises, it will feel better afterward. Exercise is definitely a good way of relieving stress. It balances out brain chemistry, so your animal can let go of any anxiety it might have.

Parts of the musculoskeletal system don't have a direct blood supply:

- Ligaments
- Tendons
- Cartilage

They get their nutrition through diffusion. That happens through compression and decompression as they move, like in the case of cartilages. The action is like a pump or like a sponge. You squeeze the sponge, then you release it. It fills back up with fluid, you squeeze it again, and it squishes the fluid out.

That's how these connective tissues get their nutrition. If they don't move, they don't get adequate nourishment. Movement also stimulates neuronal pathways. So any time an animal moves, their brain is integrating a lot of information. That's important, especially for animals who have issues with pain.

You don't want to overdo it if an animal is really uncomfortable, but the less they move, the more pain they will end up having. The input from the nervous system regarding movement inhibits some of the pain information that travels to the brain. Again, obviously, if there's a broken leg it's not a good idea to move. You have to be smart about it. Especially with something like arthritis, you have to keep the body moving a bit just so that it will inhibit some of the pain sensations.

The less your animal moves the more muscle mass it will lose and the more unstable its joints will become. If the joints are already inflamed, the degeneration and pain will only get worse.

Movement circulates lymphatic fluid. It helps with detoxification because it brings more blood flow to the liver and the kidneys. It helps with absorption of food because it stimulates appetite and better digestion, and it burns fat.

Here's How

When you exercise your friend, it's important that you do so safely. A dog chasing after a ball will make quick turns and abrupt sort of stop-and-go motions while attempting to catch the ball. Those movements can make them more prone to injuries. If this is the way you exercise your animal, I recommend aiming the ball at a bush or anything that forces them to slow down before they reach the ball.

To exercise any animal, be aware of which muscle groups they're using, and which muscle groups might be not developed as well. If your animal does a lot of exercise or sports, it's important to make sure that you balance demand on different muscle groups appropriately. For example, big dogs tend to use more of their leg muscles to move themselves. They don't engage the core musculature so much. Doing some training and balancing exercises with them will help to strengthen and activate some of the core muscles they're not using very much.

Core muscle exercises help them develop:

- Stability
- Balance
- Performance

These exercises also reduce the risk for injury.

If your animal has arthritis, you may consider giving them the opportunity to swim. While swimming, the animal is moving but doesn't have to carry its whole body weight. Cross-training is another way to give them more endurance.

With horses, the same is true. It's important that they move in a way that is physiologically appropriate so that they won't injure themselves and they don't build tension in their muscles.

When exercising and riding horses we also need to take into account their age and fitness level. Horses are not fully grown until they're at least five-and-a-half years old (older in taller individuals). That's when the growth plates in the spine close.

And isn't it exactly that part we sit on as a rider?

A little known fact is that the lower neck vertebrae close last. Thus, cranking on their necks early in their training (or ever, really) is not a good idea. Some of the bones that make the hock joint don't finish growing until they're four years old.

Could that be why we see so many hock issues in horses?

Giving any animal a chance to fully and gradually develop their physical body is crucial.

Just like with us humans, it's a matter of training for what we need. Any dancer, for example, learns to use the body appropriately and correctly to be able to perform the movements. So do our animals. They have the innate ability to move properly. But in horses, for example, if we sit on them, that's a whole different kind of balance they have to develop. It's important that we get them to move in a way that is not damaging to them, but is supportive, correct, and strengthening.

It goes without saying that as a rider you have to get proper training yourself, and make sure that your body is aligned as to not interfere with your horse.

I remember a horse who was lame and had recurrent issues at the *pol*, or the area of the first cervical vertebra. Wouldn't you know, the rider had the same issue with her neck? Once it was fixed, the horse's lameness was 90 percent improved.

Amazing, isn't it?

Everything and everybody is connected.

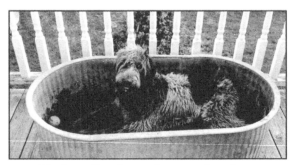
Hank, cooling down after a good workout

Questions and Action Steps

Take a lesson in dog fitness and balancing so that you can learn some exercises to do with them (see www.PeakAnimalHealthCenter.com for resources)

Provide daily exercise according to their ability.

For horses: try to extend their time outdoors, or better yet, allow them to roam 24/7. Encourage more movement by enriching their environment and adding a companion to their turnout if possible (see www.PeakAnimalHealthCenter.com for ideas).

CONCLUSION: PULLING IT ALL TOGETHER

I hope that after reading about these six pillars, you have reached an understanding that all of the parts need to work together and even more importantly, that they are dependent on one another. That's really how you need to address health and healing, because if you address only one aspect, you will not get the same results.

To briefly recap:

- You need to give your animal adequate nourishment.

- Their cells need the nutrients to be able to function properly.

- The GI tract has to be able to get the nutrients into the body.

- Detoxification must be uninterrupted to get rid of wastes and whatever is impairing the body's optimum function.

- Communication systems must be working properly via hormones and the nervous system so the cells know what to do and when to do it.

- Fitness and exercise help to increase all of the individual systems.

If you can do all of this, your animal friend will have the best chance of health and vitality. You will be able to decrease the dreaded and destructive chronic inflammatory processes that affect many animals' health and ability to enjoy life to the fullest.

CASE STORIES

Who doesn't like stories?

I live for happy endings and wish the same for you with all my heart. Hopefully the following stories will give you hope and encouragement to embark on this wonderful journey to greater health.

Jake

Jake is a thirteen-year-old Siberian husky.

He had no immediate health concerns except for "mild stiffness in his hips."

His family wanted to do everything to prevent health issues from appearing down the road.

Despite the stiffness, he still ran several miles with his people a few times a week. I put him on my Optimizing Wellness Program. We changed his diet from kibble to raw. We detoxified his body. We worked on enhancing his GI function with enzymes, probiotics and fecal transplant. He also received fish oil and chiropractic adjustments to help his mobility.

After a very short period of time his family noticed a change in his attitude and behavior. As a young dog he had been abused and even though he has been with his family for many years, he was still ducking when they tried to pet him, as if he was afraid of being beaten. With his renewed vigor he was much more confident and stopped ducking.

Do you remember how I mentioned that when you restore proper functioning that everything heals at once? That's exactly what happened with Jake and what I see every day. To this day it surprises me how the body can change.

If you give the body what it needs and take away what it doesn't need, you may be surprised by how much even a healthy animal can improve.

Bear

I met Bear because he had been diagnosed with IBD (irritable bowel disease) that caused him to have episodes of bloody diarrhea, vomiting, and lack of appetite. Even though he wasn't eating much he was gaining weight. As a five-year-old German shepherd he was also suffering from severe anxiety and pruritus (itching). To make matters more difficult, he was also diagnosed with C. difficile infection and multiple food sensitivities.

Bear was supposed to be a police dog, but his anxiety and chronic GI issues prevented him from being a good candidate. When I met him, his people had already taken several steps to help him heal, including putting him on a raw diet that excluded all the foods he was sensitive to. They also gave him digestive aids and herbs. Given that he had antibiotics for his C. diff infection and his long history of GI issues, I had a very strong suspicion that he was suffering from increased intestinal permeability (leaky gut).

Thus, the first step was to restore his GI tract to reduce overall inflammation. Microbiome Restorative Therapy (fecal transplants) worked miracles for this dog. His fecal consistency normalized almost instantaneously, his anxiety decreased significantly and he became his playful self again. In the process he was also put on a detoxification protocol and his hormonal imbalances were addressed. He suffered from a mildly sluggish thyroid gland and adrenal stress.

Just like a car with dashboard warning lights, Bear had his own pointer in the form of a scab on his nose (located at the large intestine meridian end point). Every time a new food was introduced, the owners watched to see if it lit up, so to speak. If not, it meant that he was tolerating the addition.

Going through the Wellness Program restored Bear's health to the point where everyone was feeling better and enjoying life together.

Xuxa

Xuxa, a three-and-a-half-year-old Havanese, is another example demonstrating the importance of addressing all pillars. This dog suffered from allergies since she was six months old. Her symptoms had worsened over time and the scratching was most pronounced at night. In addition she had had surgery for patellar luxation in both knees. Recovery from the second surgery had been quite difficult. Her family also noted that she had lost hair at the top of her head.

Based on lab work, Xuxa's allergies were determined to be environmental. She suffered from some minor hormonal imbalance, which was addressed with supplements. After her first chiropractic treatment, her people were surprised to see how much more lively she was.

Sometimes it is hard to see if an animal is in pain, especially if the discomfort is present in multiple areas. To restore her immune system function, she too received a GI overhaul to counteract effects of prior medication. Detoxification helped to improve liver and overall functioning of her body. In the process of uncovering her allergy mystery, we discovered that she was highly allergic to dryer sheets. Several Nambudripad Allergy Elimination Technique (NAET) treatments further assisted her immune system to respond normally to the environment. As the cherry on top of the cake, the hair on top of her head started growing again. The fuzzy face is back.

Unfortunately, when running after a ball, she tore one of her cruciate ligaments and needed surgery. After having been on antibiotics to prevent infection, she started to chew on her feet again. A simple fecal transplant to restore her gut flora took care of it. Due to being in much better health, she just flew through the recovery process at record speed.

Peppy

Peppy is an eighteen-year-old thoroughbred gelding with a two-year history of recurrent Equine Protozoal Myeltoenciphalitis (EPM) and Polyneuritis equi. When I met him, he had been on several rounds of medication to eradicate the infection. The most pronounced neurologic sign was a significant atrophy of his back muscles. A very slight gait abnormality in the rear was noted.

In addition he also showed other signs such as right hind weakness and fecal water that made me suspect leaky gut. His hind legs would swell as well as his sheath. Lack of energy was another complaint, for which he was receiving Thyro-L. Just like with the above animals we addressed all six pillars of health.

We changed Peppy's diet to provide his body with all the nutrients he needed, including supplements to heal his hind gut. Because his thyroid hormone levels were still low despite medication, we switched him to a natural thyroid hormone and added iodine. Detoxification was also part of the treatment to assist with cleaning his liver and metabolic pathways. The goal was to get his body temperature back up into the normal range (100–100.8° F). His was far too low and erratic.

Within a couple of months, his stopped having fecal water, his hind legs were stocking up much less, and his top line had rebuilt significantly. The other neurological signs disappeared and his lab values improved, indicating that the immune system attack on the nerve sheaths (polyneuritis) was diminishing.

Bravo

Bravo is a very sweet twenty-one-year-old Tennessee walking horse gelding. His main problems were weight gain, recurrent thrush, and allergies to gnats. Just like Peppy and many horses I meet, he had a body temperature below 100° F, which invites all kinds of pathogens to have a party — in his case, thrush. Thrush is not caused by dampness. Dampness can make it worse, but it is a weak immune system that is the culprit.

Have you ever wondered why it is that in the same environment some horses get thrush while others never do?

Hormone testing indicated an imbalance including low T3 and T4 as well as elevated estrogen, which is inflammatory, and a dysregulated immune system as indicated by low levels of immunoglobulins. A change in diet, detoxification, and hormone replacement helped significantly. To make him more comfortable, thrush treatment was instituted.

CHAPTER FIVE

Personal Responsibility

A HOLISTIC VIEW OF YOUR LIFE

Everything you do in life has a consequence. Often we compartmentalize. For example, you might get good nutrition — you go to a health food store and buy a lot of organic things — but the organic things are packaged in plastic or the strawberries come from Mexico or California or thousands of miles away. Yes, they're organic, but the carbon footprint they leave behind and the amount of toxins that are being produced in order to get the organic strawberries to somewhere thousands of miles away can't be ignored. Packaged, organic food will nourish your body a little bit more, but at the same time it's creating more toxicity in the environment, which your body then has to deal with.

We need to think beyond immediate comfort. Often we look for something that's comfortable and easy. I understand; I'm like that too.

We live in a busy world and we all have a lot on our plates, but we could do just a little bit more to think globally:

- Recycle
- Buy less plastic
- Use nontoxic cleaning products
- Keep things simple

We can achieve a lot by taking some very simple steps.

Choices for a Healthy Environment

It's great if you can feed your animal raw food or species-appropriate food that's good quality, but if you use a lot of chemicals around the house or you store their food in plastic, you are counteracting that. Your immune system and your animal's immune system get compromised by all of these toxins.

As an example, if you have been using antibacterial soaps, consider giving them up, because microbes have a lot of good functions; killing the good with the bad can cause problems. Focusing on you and your family for a moment, studies have found that children growing up on farms and around animals tend to have fewer allergies and asthma. Thankfully, there's a reversing trend of going back to our roots and how things used to be, which works better than a lot of that modern technology. Eating a little bit of dirt everyday gives you some probiotics and helps your immune system.

You can rethink your lifestyle choices and become more conscious of the difference those choices make for you, your family, your animals, and our beautiful Mother Earth. It's not about being perfect. We don't live in a perfect world. Just do as much as you can to contribute in a good way. You can reuse plastic bags, or use canvas bags that don't break and can be used over and over again. Simple little things like that can make a big difference in the long run.

Wolves at Yellowstone

We humans are the biggest destructive pests on this planet. Mostly, when we humans interfere with something, it backfires. There is one example I mentioned earlier in which human intervention did turn out well, and that was the reintroduction of wolves to Yellowstone National Park.

In 1995, after a seventy-year absence, wolves were reintroduced into Yellowstone. Their presence changed the entire ecosystem there, including the animals. Some of the animals that were there in abundance were reduced in numbers, and others were able to thrive. More birds returned. Different kinds of birds, different kinds of animals, and different kinds of plants were able to take root again.

Erosion decreased because more plants were growing. Birds were spreading seeds via their droppings. Because there was less soil erosion and more vegetation, the river started to meander less. It changed the way the river was flowing, because everything changed. That was just because of the introduction of the wolves. Maybe it worked because their presence was a return to how things had been before.

If we return to the foods and more natural lifestyles that used to be part of our ancestry — especially for animals — then we have a much better chance at returning animals, ourselves, and the whole planet back to a healthier state, too. With every being that feels better, we increase the well-being and consciousness of the entire planet. The consciousness of the planet will change to having a much better vibration. That's what we all need! We need to change so that we can heal.

HONESTLY ASSESS YOUR ROLE AS YOUR ANIMAL'S CAREGIVER

The best way to predict the future is to create it.
~ Author unknown

How Willing Are You?

How important is it to resolve your animal's issues?

How willing are you to provide them with what they need to have the happiest life possible?

As a guardian of your animals, you are responsible for their health and their well-being. You are also their advocates. Don't be afraid to stand up for them and don't let yourself be pushed into anything that doesn't feel right. Do your research. Listen to your gut and intuition. It is likely your animal speaking to you.

Taking Action

If you want things to change — if you want your animals to be healthier, if you want whatever symptoms they have to go away — you must take action. Unless you take action, nothing will change. You can gather all the information you need, but unless you use it, nothing will happen. Einstein said that the definition of insanity is doing the same thing over and over again, expecting a different result. Even if it's just a small action step that you can take today, I encourage you to take it, because it will eventually build up to become bigger and bigger. You may be very surprised by how things evolve.

It does not necessarily require taking huge leaps. Little steps will keep you from getting overwhelmed. If I try to do too much at once, I end up overwhelmed and I don't do anything. Choose things that can be easily done and fit into your life. Then, once you become accustomed to that change, something else can be added.

Take small steps. When your animal is sick, of course, you'll need to do a bigger intervention. Nevertheless, it's not something that has to be big and difficult.

When I work with people, I keep it simple. I keep treatment and follow-up easy so that it's doable and doesn't take a lot of additional time. By changing things a little bit, you can make big strides, especially if you change them in the right way by addressing the Six Pillars described in Chapter Four.

The saying, "An ounce of prevention is worth a pound of cure," is very true and is a guideline that everybody should follow when it comes to health.

Living a long, happy, healthy life is much better than living a mediocre life or a life of poor health quality just because we didn't take care of it early enough. Issues bubble under the surface, then they pop up as a big symptom and we wonder about it.

"How did that happen?" we wonder.

Or you might come down with something "all of the sudden," which is usually not true—it's usually something that has been building up over time.

You need to make sure that you keep your animal's body functioning well, because they really need it. It's just like caring for your own body. Think about the care you put into making sure your car is in good shape: You get it into service; you get new tires; you do all sorts of things to keep it running. If your car isn't working well, you have a problem.

You need to do the same thing for your animals. You need to give them healthy food, provide exercise, maintain their nervous system, and detoxify their system. You need to do all of these things in order to maintain their bodies.

SELF-LOVE AND REVERENCE FOR EVERYTHING

It is not my intention to make you feel bad about what you have or haven't done. You are where you are on the spectrum of learning how to provide the best for your animal. It's a journey for you and your animals. You chose that journey to learn what you need to learn. My job is to support you in your journey and teach you.

If you are judging yourself harshly, try to accept where you are on your journey and find forgiveness for yourself. Your animals are definitely not judging you. Animals love us no matter what; whether we feed them crappy food or not. They love us. Obviously they would love to have a good life, too–just like anyone else–but it's about finding forgiveness and acceptance for where we are, and forgive our ignorance. Once we have gained more knowledge, it is our responsibility to make use of it.

I hear from a lot of people, "If I had only known," or, "I wish I knew; I would have done it better."

I have found myself thinking these things as well. You learn from all of your experiences. If you learn from it and try to do better, that's really all that's needed and all that matters. Hopefully you won't repeat the same mistakes, but use what you learn, move on, and do better.

Gratitude

If you view everything with a softer eye or through the lens of forgiveness, you can find a lot of gratitude for what you've gone through and what you've learned from your animals or with your animals. That makes it easier to deal with conflicts as well. With gratitude for all that you've gone through, for your journey, it's easier to find forgiveness for the things that you do and the mistakes that you think you might have made.

Even if it may not look like it in this moment, your journey is really perfect. Find reverence for it. It's all perfect in some way or another. Sometimes we don't know that until several years later.

APPENDIX

ADDITIONAL CONSIDERATIONS FOR OPTIMAL HEALTH

Here are a few miscellaneous subjects that are also crucial for maximizing your animal's health. They are important to investigate in order to make the best choices for your animal.

Teeth

Teeth and the mouth serve many functions:

- Chewing
- Swallowing
- Tearing plants from the ground
- Pulling meat off of a carcass

The health of the mouth is not just about the ability to chew and process food. A problem in the mouth—for instance, gingivitis in a dog or a cat—can cause problems throughout the body:

- It can affect the information going to the brain.

- Bacteria from the mouth can travel through the bloodstream to other areas such as the heart.

- Alignment of the teeth can affect the structural alignment of the rest of the body.

The whole mouth is highly innervated and provides a lot of proprioceptive information into the brain. *Proprioception* means knowing where the body is in space. For that reason and many others, it's important that the mouth be healthy.

The teeth also play a role in sound body structure. Horses are particularly prone to dental misalignment. This can result from misuse of a bit for riding, poor dental work, or trauma. As a result, it can cause them to lose their back musculature. They can trip more. The issues can intensify as we sit on horse, urge them to go at rather high speeds, ask them to carry us while they jump, and perform movements that require very good balance.

You must make sure that the dental balance is established properly, so that you decrease the risk of injuries and falls. Additionally, the animal is much more comfortable when the teeth are aligned. A misaligned bite can feel like a kernel of corn stuck between your teeth; it's very uncomfortable and very annoying. In some horses I have treated, their mouth troubles have caused headaches, stomach pains, and other issues.

I often hear owners say, "I want somebody to float my horse's teeth without sedation."

That's a fine choice, but if your horse is not cooperating, the vet or equine dentist cannot do a proper job. Sedating or not sedating should not be the determining factor for which equine dentist you hire. It should be based on the dentist's ability to correctly balance your horse's teeth.

When you clean your dog's or cat's teeth without sedation, it is impossible to do a thorough job. It may work if they just have a little bit of tartar stuck on one of their teeth; you can just pop it off. But if their whole mouth is full of tartar, they will likely also need radiographs to evaluate the health and viability of the teeth and their roots.

Teeth can be a source of chronic infection and therefore persistently affect the body, just as in human medicine. For example, for certain people having a root canal can be very detrimental to health, because there is a constant release of toxins from bacteria living in the dead tooth.

It's necessary to clean the tartar from animals' teeth. Providing them with species-appropriate nutrition and a raw bone to chew on, their teeth can remain white as pearls into their old age.

Teeth are an inside job. Feed your dog right, make sure they don't have inflammation in their body, give them a bone to chew on once in a while, and that should really take care of it. Of course you can brush their teeth, too; that is definitely an option. I don't recommend putting any kind of anti-plaque products into their drinking water. If they don't like the taste, they might become dehydrated.

More information on how to keep teeth healthy and the mouth functional can be found on my website, www. PeakAnimalHealthCenter.com.

Parasites:

> *Vital animals don't get parasites.*
> ~ Will Falconer

Generally, the sicker the animal, the more likely they are to have parasites and to attract parasites. Parasites such as fleas, heartworm, and tapeworms are trying to survive, so they're not trying to kill the host. If they kill their host, they die as well. Creating better health will help with that issue. If parasites are present, it could indicate other ways in which your animal's health is compromised.

Heartworm

A lot of vaccinations and medications that are prescribed for diseases or conditions are really driven by fear. That's part of the marketing strategy that is used. Heartworm is one example, especially in some of the northern areas of the country.

We need to look at the facts. For one, there's no heartworm transmission possible when temperature goes below 57° F. The larval development of a mosquito has stopped. At 64° F it takes approximately one month for the mosquito larvae to become infectious.

Guess how long a mosquito lives?

Three to four weeks.

There are different requirements necessary for the transmission of heartworm to even occur outside of optimal temperature. The mosquito needs to be female and of a particular species. The female mosquito must have fed off of an infected animal in order to transfer heartworm.

Heartworm (and flea and tick) preventatives are not without risk; they can cause:

- Liver problems
- Vomiting
- Diarrhea
- Loss of appetite
- Depression
- Lethargy
- Skin eruptions
- Seizures

- Tremors
- Paralysis
- Autoimmune disorders
- Thyroid problems
- Fever
- Weakness
- Dizziness
- Coughing
- Nose bleeds
- Difficulty breathing
- Pneumonia
- Irritability
- Sudden aggressive behavior
- Nerve damage
- Fertility problems
- Sudden death

Very often the side effects don't show up until ten to fourteen days after the monthly product was given and typically starts after an animal has had two to five doses. Occasionally signs can develop after your animal has been on a preventative for a long time.

Vaccines

Unless you live under a rock you are probably aware of the vaccine controversy. Vaccines—as protective as they may be—come with an array of potential adverse reactions. Studies have shown that many vaccines provide long-term and even life-long protection, making yearly boosters unnecessary and potentially dangerous to your beloved friend.

The American Animal Hospital Association (AAHA) changed their recommendations for vaccinations to every three (or even more) years for dogs, yet many veterinarians are not up to date on that knowledge. Over-vaccination places undue stress on the immune system, in some cases causing it to attack the body's own tissue, to the point of being life-threatening.

Health issues that can arise due to over-vaccination include:

- Immune-mediated hemolytic anemia (IMHA)
- Immune-related thrombocytopenia
- Neurological disorders
- Encephalitis
- Liver and kidney failure
- Autoimmune thyroiditis
- Malignant vaccine-related tumors
- Laminitis and colic in horses
- Allergies
- Behavior changes
- Heart failure
- Lameness
- Screaming pain
- Fever

- Polyarthritis
- Dermatitis
- Uncontrollable itching
- Pancreatitis
- Mast cell disease
- Urinary tract infections
- Diarrhea
- Seizures
- Chronic weight loss
- Enlarged spleen
- Cancer
- Death

Please make sure that you're well informed of the pros and cons of each vaccine. I see far too many animals with serious vaccine injuries.

A very simple solution to check your animal's protection from life-threatening infectious diseases is *titer testing*.

Titer testing

A titer test is a blood test that measures the amount of antibodies present to fight a specific disease, such as:

- Distemper
- Feline panleukopenia
- Rabies
- Tetanus

- Equine herpes virus
- West Nile virus

Titers accurately assess an animal's protection and help veterinarians judge the need for booster vaccinations. All animals can have titers tested. For more information, visit www.PeakAnimalHealthCenter.com/vaccines-and-titer-testing/.

Vaccination Rules:

IF YOUR ANIMAL IS NOT HEALTHY, DO NOT VACCINATE!

Even if it is more convenient because you're already at the vet, it is a bad idea to vaccinate an animal that is sick, was sedated, or put under anesthesia or just had surgery, even if it is dental cleaning.

Don't let convenience and saving a few dollars dictate your actions. Do what is best for your animal, because vaccines are not harmless. They can cause a lot of adverse effects.

Unfortunately, many veterinarians ignore this very important rule, even though it can be found on every vaccine insert. Be your animals' advocates. They need you.

So, again the number one rule of vaccination: Do not vaccinate if your animal is not healthy!

In the case of rabies, even though it is the law to vaccinate your dogs, many states allow vaccine exemptions for rabies if the animal isn't healthy.

Conclusion

As you've been reading through this book, I'm sure it has become very clear to you that preventive care is the best gift you can give your animal and yourself. Instead of waiting for advanced disease to set in, start to maximize your friend's health today. It's doable!

I want to see smiles on your animal's face and yours. I want suffering to end and watch animals live their lives with a spring in their step and with the joy that comes from feeling well.

Please help make this happen and share with your friends and family what you've learned from reading this book. They might be looking for a solution too. Let's change the world of *disease*-care to one of *health*-care together.

Thank you for reading my book. I look forward to hearing about your successes and am here to help if you need it.

Next Steps

Here are a few suggestions of what you can do right now to improve your animal's health:

1. Feed your animal a species-appropriate diet. It can be bought from a store, premade, frozen in patties that are easy to take out, or in bags for horses that are also easy to put in a bucket. You can also go a little bit further and make the food yourself. You can find recipes and recommendations for balanced diets, especially for dogs and cats, in a lot of good books. Less information is available for horses, but more information can also be found on my website, www.PeakAnimalHealthCenter.com.

2. Read labels: Check products you are feeding your animals, using around the house, and using on your animals. Look at the list of ingredients; keep it to things that you know and that you can pronounce. My philosophy for shampoos, for example is that I don't buy any shampoo that has ingredients I don't recognize. If I don't know what it is, I don't buy it. Do a little bit of research to find products that are more environmentally friendly and nontoxic for your own animals. They can be found at different health food

stores. Regular stores are carrying natural brands more and more. Just be careful about the words "natural" or "green" being used on some of these products, because they often still contain harmful chemicals. The Environmental Working Group is a good resource to check if your products are safe: www.ewg.org.

3. Research vaccines. Limit the amount of vaccines that you're using by doing titer testing. There's more information on my website about that.

4. Take a breath together. Maybe meditate together once in a while, or spend some time out in nature with your animal, just enjoying the smells, sounds, and colors.

5. Keep learning. If you don't know something, or if you want more information on something your regular veterinarian recommends, ask them or ask someone who knows. Do some research online. Go to my website and send me an email; I'd be more than happy to help you if you need information on a subject.

Image Credits

Page 27 Image credit: Pixabay

Page 43 Image credits:

Wilting gerbera plant: dreamstime
Sun: http://clipartfreefor.com/files/4/87337.html
Bug: http://www.pd4pic.com/smile/7/
Warning sign: http://all-free-download.com/free-vector/download/sign_toxic_clip_art_16661.html
Watering can: http://all-free-download.com/free-vector/vector-watering-can.html

Page 52 Image credit: Dreamstime

Page 53 Image credit:

For publishing and copyright info:
https://openi.nlm.nih.gov/detailedresult.php?img=PMC3121438_1838fig2&req=4

Page 54 Image credits:

Water fountain, environmental pollution image, capsule, dog food, farmer: Pixabay.
Corncob, Chemicals/msg: Pixabay and Suter;
Rabbit: from http://www.clipartof.com/download?download_id=
a7280e9999696b2d34f3e82d0f9cd1bc

Dog: Flickr/Mr TGT, Creative Commons license (http://phys.org/news/2013-01-dog-life-friend-fattest.html)

Page 78 Image credit: Suter

Page 85 Image credit: Suter

Page 97 Image credit:

Golden Dollar sign from http://www.clipartbest.com/clipart-eiM8GbKin

Page 98 Image credit:

Copyright © Return2Health Limited. All Rights Reserved.

Page 106 Image credit:

Liver and GI: Pixabay
Dog: Copyright © PETS ADVISOR (modified)

Page 114 Image credit:

Printed with permission from Dr. Josh Axe at www.draxe.com

Page 119 Image credit:

Doggie Heaven Hotel Blog: http://www.doggieheavenhotel.com/2013/06/

Page 121 Image credits:

Donkey and Coins: Pixabay
Money bag: http://www.clipartbest.com/clipart-LTKzxnyTa

Page 128 Image credit:
Dog and Lungs: Pixabay

Page 130 Image credit: Suter

Page 144 Image credit: Suter

About the Author

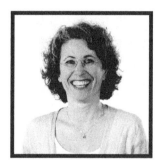

Dr. Odette Suter, DVM, is a holistic veterinarian and educator to animal caretakers and veterinarians alike.

Early in her studies, she recognized the limitations of conventional medicine and questioned its role in true healing. Thus began the search into holistic and functional medicine, including Chinese Medicine, Veterinary Spinal Manipulation and Chiropractic Neurology, Applied Kinesiology, NAET, Animal Communication, and Nutrition, with the goal to have the tools to address all aspects of being.

Focusing on quality versus quantity and prevention rather than Band-aids, Dr. Suter utilizes functional medicine principles to address the essential keys to resolving the underlying stressors that lead to disease.

Her own healing journey has led her to explore many avenues of healing, which she has integrated into her veterinary practice.

With her passion for teaching, Dr. Suter has created an intensive educational program for her clients to teach them how to create longevity for their animals and empower them to know how to maintain their companion's health.

Visit her website at www.PeakAnimalHealthCenter. com.

Medicine is not only a science; it is also an art. It does not consist of compounding pills and plasters; it deals with the very processes of life, which must be understood before they may be guided.

~ Paracelsus

Made in the USA
Las Vegas, NV
13 January 2024

84316048R00105